CLINICAL
EPIDEMIOLOGY

THE SCIENTIST'S LIBRARY
Biology and Medicine

EDITED BY
PETER P. H. DE BRUYN, M.D.

Experimental Design and Its Statistical Basis
D. J. Finney
(1955)

Aggression
John Paul Scott
(1958)

Bone
Franklin C. McLean and Marshall R. Urist
(Rev. ed., 1961)

The Biochemistry of Intracellular Parasitism
James W. Moulder
(1962)

The Evolution of the Human Brain
Gerhardt Von Bonin
(1963)

The Fossil Evidence for Human Evolution
W. E. Le Gros Clark
(Rev. ed., 1964)

Clinical Epidemiology
John R. Paul
(Rev. ed., 1966)

CLINICAL
EPIDEMIOLOGY

BY

JOHN R. PAUL

Revised Edition

THE UNIVERSITY OF CHICAGO PRESS

Chicago and London

Library of Congress Catalog Card Number: 66–13883

THE UNIVERSITY OF CHICAGO PRESS, CHICAGO & LONDON
The University of Toronto Press, Toronto 5, Canada
© *1958, 1966 by The University of Chicago*

Dedicated to the memory
of
two former friends and colleagues—
Leslie T. Webster, M.D.
(1894–1943)
and
James D. Trask, M.D.
(1890–1942)
both epidemiologists, in experimental
and clinical fields, respectively

Preface to the Series

During the past few decades the investigative approaches to biological problems have become markedly diversified. This diversification has been caused in part by the introduction of methods from other fields, such as mathematics, physics, and chemistry, and in part has been brought about by the formulation of new problems within biology. At the same time, the quantity of scientific production and publication has increased. Under these circumstances, the biologist has to focus his attention more and more exclusively on his own field of interest. This specialization, effective as it is in the pursuit of individual problems, requiring ability and knowledge didactically unrelated to biology, is detrimental to a broad understanding of the current aspects of biology as a whole, without which conceptual progress is difficult.

The purpose of "The Scientist's Library: Biology and Medicine" series is to provide authoritative information about the growth and status in various areas in such a fashion that the individual books may be read with profit not only by the specialist but also by those whose interests lie in other fields. The topics for the series have been selected as representative of active fields of science, especially those that have developed markedly in recent years as the result of new methods and new discoveries.

The textual approach is somewhat different from that ordinarily used by the specialist. The authors have been asked to emphasize introductory concepts and problems, and the present status of their subjects, and to clarify terminology and methods of approach instead of limiting themselves to detailed accounts of current factual knowledge. The authors have also been asked to assume a common level of scientific competence rather than to attempt popularization of the subject matter.

Consequently, the books should be of interest and value to workers in the various fields of biology and medicine. For the teacher and investigator, and for students entering specialized areas, they will provide familiarity with the aims, achievements, and present status of these fields.

PETER P. H. DE BRUYN

Chicago, Illinois

Preface to the Revised Edition

In presenting a review of epidemiology, I have tried in this revision, as in the first edition, to avoid the inclusion of too many technical details or the introduction of too much sophistication into the subject. In a swiftly moving field such as this one, with new ideas and methods coming along all the time, one can easily err on the side of introducing too many new and complicated methods and of attempting to be too erudite. On the other hand, one can readily err by attempting to achieve simplicity that actually becomes naivete. Indeed one can easily simplify away from the truth because it is easier to use short cuts instead of complicated explanations.

As in the previous edition many of the chapters have been taken from lectures given to medical students. Some of them represent the basis of a course of instruction, which has been variously entitled "Principles of Epidemiology," or "Clinical Epidemiology." This course has been offered, since 1945 at Yale University partly to medical students or as an introduction to public health students. Understandably its context has undergone great changes within the past dozen years.

Epidemiology has often been regarded as a discipline useful only to those engaged in public health activities, or in schools of hygiene, or departments or ministries of health. One may ask then why medical students or physicians should be concerned with it, particularly since their busy hours of work and reading are so taken up already. Of the various answers that one might give to this question a primary one is that more and more authors of textbooks of internal medicine have come to recognize the importance of including a section on epidemiology, if a modern description of a given disease is to be complete. Another is that as preventive medicine comes increasingly to the fore, an awareness has developed that epidemiology stands today in somewhat the same relationship to that subject as do some of the more familiar basic medical sciences to curative medicine. Anatomy, pathology, microbiology, physiology, and pharmacology are all considered basic and introductory to the study of disease processes and to the clinical care of patients; in like manner the concept of epidemiology, as presented here, can at least substitute as one of these "preclinical" subjects. A concept concerned with the circumstances under which a person or people get sick or remain sick is basic to any attempt to alter these circumstances so as to protect individuals from future illness. Thus preventive medicine is, in this sense, applied epidemiology. It is this which has brought the epidemiological aspect of medicine increasingly to the fore as part of the modern physician's academic job.

For a variety of reasons the scope of this book has many inadequacies and obviously falls far short of orthodox concepts of epidemiology which are taught in schools of hygiene or public health in this country and probably elsewhere. There the subject is usually presented in a much broader form illustrated by large populations, and also with far more emphasis on epidemiology as a statistical science. Such is not the purpose of this small volume. It is not exactly a primer, but its purpose, as already expressed, is to introduce the subject to doctors or students of medicine, biologists, sociologists, or others, in semi-technical terms and with examples they might use. Thus the book is for those who consider themselves amateur human ecologists, or perhaps for "epidemiological clinicians." In particular, it is for clinical investigators. It is not for those whose interests are preeminently statistical.

Another deficiency may be that the approach suffers from being too heavily weighted with examples of infectious disease with a relative neglect of non-infectious conditions. This selection of topics has been done advisedly, for as was stated in the first edition of this text, this book is meant to be an introduction to the subject, and it is easier to begin with infectious disease.

Nevertheless, the conditions usually regarded as non-infectious have received more attention in this second edition; for instance, besides coronary artery disease, the epidemiology of carcinoma and particularly carcinoma of the lung have been included.

For assistance in the preparation of the text as well as for valuable criticism I am greatly indebted to the following colleagues at the Yale University School of Medicine: Dr. Anthony M-M. Payne, Dr. Lloyd Stevenson, Dr. Colin M. White, Dr. Wilbur G. Downs, Dr. Richard M. Taylor, Dr. Jack Henderson, and Dr. Alvan R. Feinstein; and to Dr. Margaret J. Albrink, Morgantown, W.Va.; Dr. Oglesby Paul, Chicago, Ill.; and Dr. Michael B. Shimkin, Philadelphia, Pa. And for similar assistance, as well as that of preparing the indexes of both the first and second edition texts and helping in other ways, I owe much to Dr. Dorothy M. Horstmann and Dr. Robert M. McCollum.

I also wish to acknowledge the assistance of Mr. Armin Hemberger and Miss Virginia Simon for preparing some of the illustrations and that of Mrs. Raymond Fitch, Mrs. Harry Wenzel, and my wife for typing parts of the manuscript.

I am also indebted to the following agencies and publishing companies: the American Cancer Society, New York, N.Y.; the California State Board of Health, San Francisco, Calif.; the *Journal of the American Medical Association*, Chicago, Ill.; the J. B. Lippincott Company, Philadelphia, Pa.; E. & S. Livingstone Ltd., Edinburgh, Scotland; the *Yale Journal of Biology and Medicine*, New Haven, Conn.; and finally to the U.S. Public Health Service for its kind permission to reproduce certain tables and illustrations from its Surveillance Reports furnished by the Communicable Disease Center, Atlanta, Ga., and for certain other courtesies.

JOHN R. PAUL

New Haven, Connecticut

Preface to the First Edition

Epidemiology has usually been regarded as a discipline useful only to those engaged in public health activities, either in schools of hygiene or public health or in departments or ministries of health, municipal, state, or national. One may ask then why a practicing physician or any physician should be concerned with it, particularly since his busy hours of work and his reading are so overcrowded already. Of the various answers that one might give to this question, a primary one is that epidemiology stands today in somewhat the same relationship to the practice of *preventive medicine* as do some of the more familiar basic medical sciences to *curative medicine*. Pathology, pathologic physiology, and pharmacology are basic and introductory to the clinical care of patients; in like manner the concept of epidemiology, as presented here—a science concerned with the *circumstances* under which a person or persons get sick or remain sick—is basic to any attempt to alter these circumstances so as to protect individuals from future illness. In this new sense physicians certainly have a place in this field. Indeed the last ten years have seen a growing familiarity by clinicians with epidemiologic methods as applied to the behavior of a variety of diseases, both infectious and noninfectious. One could make a long list of examples: tuberculosis, coronary artery disease, and carcinoma of the lung, to name a few. Each has its epidemiologic aspect.

As for the scope of this book, it has inadequacies, and it obviously falls far short of the orthodox concept of epidemiology taught in schools of hygiene or public health in this country or elsewhere. There the subject is usually presented in a much broader form and often as a statistical science dealing with large groups of people and utilizing special mathematical methods. Such is not the purpose of this small volume. It is not exactly a primer, but its purpose is to *introduce* this subject to doctors or students of medicine, biology, or sociology in non-technical language and with examples they might use. Another deficiency may be that the approach is too heavily weighted with examples drawn from the field of infectious disease, with a relative neglect of noninfectious diseases. This selection of topics has been done advisedly. As stated above, the book is essentially an introduction to our subject, and it is easier to begin with infectious disease.

The idea of presenting in book form a review of epidemiology came from Dr. Peter P. H. De Bruyn of the University of Chicago, who has given much helpful advice. Many of the chapters have been taken from previous papers or lectures by the author, and some of them represent the basis of a course of instruction originally entitled "Principles of Epidemiology," currently called "Clinical Epidemiology," which has been given as an elective at Yale University over the past dozen years, both to public health students and to medical students.

For help in the preparation of the text, particularly on the statistical side, I am indebted for valuable criticism to Dr. Colin White, associate professor of biometry of the Department of Public Health, Yale University School of Medicine. Thanks are due also to my colleagues Dr. Dorothy M. Horstmann and Dr. Richard M. Taylor, both of the Section of Epidemiology and Preventive Medicine, Yale University School of Medicine.

I also wish to acknowledge the assistance of Mr. Armin Hemberger and Miss Sigrid Angerer for preparing some of the illustrations, and that of Mrs. Mara Iwan, Mrs. Renee Reidy, and my wife for typing parts of the manuscript.

JOHN R. PAUL

New Haven, Connecticut

Contents

Contents

APPENDIXES

INDEX

Figures

Figures

Tables

PART I

*Principles, Definitions,
and History*

CHAPTER I

Definitions and Attitudes

I shall be cautious when it comes to giving definitions of epidemiology. Broad statements are safer. Indeed, one that will do here is that modern epidemiology is *a technique whereby one explores human ecology—generally the ecology of human disease.* Clinical epidemiology focuses upon those aspects of the technique which are of immediate interest to some few physicians and clinical investigators.

DEFINITIONS

If we consult certain dictionaries, we find the term epidemiology defined as "the branch of medicine that investigates the causes and control of epidemics" (*Webster's New World Dictionary,* 1957). In others we find it defined as "the study of occurrence and distribution of disease; usually restricted to epidemic and endemic, but sometimes broadened to include all types of disease" (*Blakiston's Medical Dictionary,* 1949). The former description is today outmoded. The latter approaches the concept developed here, but it would be more adequate if it also implied that modern epidemiology deals essentially with the "ecology of disease in all its various aspects."

Actually this liberal concept of epidemiology originated 50 years ago when Dr. William H. Welch reminded us that epidemiology could include the study of the natural history of a disease (Welch 1916, p. 415) and was one of the basic sciences of preventive medicine. Supplementing this concept, Dr. W. H. Frost, one of this country's most distinguished epidemiologists, pointed out that an epidemic was only "a temporary phase in the occurrence of any disease" (Frost 1928a).

3

A broad definition of epidemiology [1] used by the author for the past three decades states that epidemiology is concerned with measurements of *the circumstances under which diseases occur, where diseases tend to flourish, and where they do not* (Paul 1938). Such circumstances may be microbiological or toxicological; they may be based on genetic, social, or environmental factors; even religious or political factors may come under scrutiny, provided they are found to have some bearing upon disease prevalence. Some of these factors may lend themselves to analysis and study within laboratories of the medical sciences, others may not.

In keeping with the idea that the term "epidemiology" goes beyond infectious disease, we may say that all diseases, all human blights and injuries, have their epidemiology—cancer, benzol poisoning, alcoholism, drug addiction, automobile accidents, suicides, and so on. Epidemiology is thus concerned with what is known or unknown about how these human ills come to pass, how they spread, what external and internal factors are responsible for them, which of these factors may be measured and—if one is fortunate enough—interpreted. Actually this approach to human ecology need not always deal with blights; it applies equally well to situations involving populations generally—even to business.

Perhaps a point of major emphasis should be that epidemiology deals with circumstances involving more than one person, a group of people upon whom something has been thrust (*epi* plus *demos*) —although the group may be no larger than a family, the inhabitants of a rooming house, or a small community—something presumably undesirable but not necessarily so. Such circumstances require some other form of expression than the mere series of cases that clinicians ordinarily use. They require the use of rates. To obtain a rate it follows that one must estimate the size

---

[1] The unqualified term "epidemiology" usually applies to human populations but epidemiology can be and should be extended to cover the animal and plant kingdoms. There is, however, special terminology for this; epizootic, for instance, refers usually to an outbreak of disease among animals.

of the group; in other words, we must determine the denominator, as well as the number of individuals affected within this group, the numerator.

Occupying a place on the periphery, as far as this book is concerned, is the applied use of this science. This concerns decisions on what to do about the findings or how to alter circumstances so as to prevent or stop the blights. Here we are getting into another field. It has already been mentioned that applied epidemiology comes under the heading of preventive medicine and the care of the public health (Welch 1916, Leavell and Clark 1958). Both concepts have their place. The applied epidemiologist's duties are like those of a fireman whose prime function is to put out fires, but the duties of the epidemiologist we speak of here, are more academic and like those who attempt to find out how conflagrations start, smolder along, or spread.

Over the years various names for what might be called clinical epidemiology have been proposed. Geographical pathology, in the sense in which this term was used by August Hirsch of Berlin almost a century ago, was one. Social medicine, another old and familiar term, covers almost too many features. Survey medicine, ecologic medicine, or community medicine have been suggested. Other terms have been social pathology, first employed by Grotjahn (1869–1931) of Berlin, and subsequently widely employed by the late Professor Ryle of the Institute of Social Medicine at Oxford (1948*a*, 1948*b*, 1949); and population pathology, used by Gordon (1955). This gives one a goodly number of terms to choose from, and yet none of them quite fills the bill, it seems to me.

Professor Ryle (1948*b*), distinguished physician that he was, visualized an evolution of medicine and described this discipline as "those environmental, domestic, occupational, economic, habitual and nutritional factors without which the intimate (or specific) causal factors of disease cannot find their opportunity" (Ryle 1948*a*). Professor Ryle, who I believe was well ahead of his time, felt that these new dimensions included a search for causes of disease which might extend well beyond the physician's examining room, certainly beyond the laboratory workbench. In view of the great and understandable stress laid today upon the importance of laboratory work and of measurements that can be carried out only in hospitals, it may be difficult for the student to appreciate that equally important clinical information can be gleaned from many other sources, as most wise and experienced physicians know. Such a discipline would employ entirely new dimensions from those ordinarily used in the orthodox practice of medicine today. And yet I believe that the number of epidemiologically minded clinicians, though always small, will materially increase.

Ecology, of course, represents the relations between organisms and their environments. Thus the concept of human ecology is probably more familiar to biologists, anthropologists, and even sociologists than to physicians, whose interests lean more toward curing sick people who are in bed than toward studying the relationships between people and their environment. But it has been true in the past and should be true in the future that among doctors there have always been naturalists—or those with something of the naturalist in them—concerned with the eternal struggles of living things to survive, be they bacteria, viruses, or men. In the past half-century at least, medical ecology has had no dearth of champions of high caliber. And by this I mean not merely a good old-fashioned college biology teacher, admirable as many of them may have been regardless of their ignorance of the molecular biology, that we take such pride in today. I mean men capable of interpreting contemporaneous scientific thought and methods about the natural history of disease, men whose vision extended beyond the limits of the usual medical scientist's workbench: Theobald Smith in the United States (1934); Charles Nicolle of Tunis (1939), the French philosopher and scientist; his friend professor Hans Zinsser of the United States, whose name might also be mentioned (1940); and Sir MacFarlane Burnet of Australia (1940, 1953). Their philosophy, dealing as it did with infectious disease, may sound out of date, but what I am speaking of is really ageless. All these men have made a strong case for the biologically and philosophically minded scientist. Even in this space age, when man considers himself more completely in charge of the world than ever before, and with his computers and new knowledge of molecular biology, more omniscient, the statement of Dr. Peyton Rous of the Rockefeller Institute (1938), made a generation ago, still holds. He reminded us then that "it is no accident that so many medical students have ranged the fields as boys for rocks and plants," for the sheer joy of it. Or that John Hunter retained this interest throughout his professional life, at the zenith of his London practice taking time to inquire into the structure and economy of whales.

Joseph Wood Krutch, the retired drama critic, though not an epidemiologist as far as I know, has been quite vocal in commenting about how lucky those people are who, whatever they do, are able to preserve in youth and adult life the joy and aura of mystery which can pervade the study of living things (1964). His plea is for the preservation of an amateur status in this field, particularly because it permits one "to speculate more freely than the specialist fearful of his responsibility dares to go." It reminds me of the sentiments of Major Greenwood of London, one of the greatest of biostatistical epidemiologists, who said in the preface of a small volume by Dr. Pickles on "Epidemiology in Country Practice" (1939): "Even in epidemiology we must have 'experts' of different kinds than amateurs and the mere fact that they are experts deprives them of many fruitful opportunities."

Such sentiments are seldom to be found in a book which attempts to propound a science and explain techniques. The clinical epidemiologist will soon enough become embroiled in problems that he will attempt to solve by all the scientific methods he can muster, and he will be encouraged—even exhorted—in the following chapters to do just this; but he must always be ready for those surprises with certain features that will remain among the incomprehensible ways which nature has of doing things. He should not always seek materialistic explanations. Why for instance, among the countless examples one might choose, has nature struck upon so complex a cycle of infecting man with a parasitic disease known as schistosomiasis? This

7

disease—with its unpronouncable name—is rare in the United States, except among Puerto Ricans, and yet it is a disease which infects countless thousands of people around the world, in Africa, Asia, and Latin America. The cycle of infestation begins with the dissemination of the eggs of the parasite in a water course, often an irrigation ditch, where there must be a special kind of snail for the development of one of the larval stages of the parasite. Subsequently, another larval stage (the cercarial stage) emerges from the snail and is then ready to penetrate the skin of that child or adult who happens to be playing or working in the irrigation ditch at that time. The adult parasite then develops in the body of the individual and goes on to produce a parasitic disease—sometimes mild, sometimes serious. It is often associated at its end stages with cancer. These are the imponderables reminding us that, regardless of man's extraordinary power and achievements, nature has infinite ways of doing things in a more or less unpredictable fashion. But this is too big a problem for us now and I do not have to emphasize that there is far more to the study of human ecology than being either an amateur or professional naturalist.

The physician or "social ecologist" is also likely to have some sympathy with man's lot from a socioeconomic standpoint. Sometimes this can erase every trace of the biologist in him, which is a pity. Yet in support of this cause we might do no better here than to hark back to the prophetic words of the late Henry S. Sigerist (1946): "That medicine is a social science sounds like a truism, yet it cannot be repeated often enough because in medical education we still act as if medicine were a natural science and nothing else." The physician has a joint moral responsibility in both fields, which some call the microcosm and the macrocosm. Indeed, almost at once, the epidemiologist must become engaged in a concern with the social cosmos, based on a system that man himself has created. The microcosm (or what I have chosen to call in this book man's microclimate) is the immediate and intimate environment, ways of living, and their effects on man's social consciousness—truly a part of man himself. A major part of the macrocosm can also be interpreted in the light of social and political philosophy and its economic structure from which neither the practice of medicine, nor medicine itself, nor the epidemiologist can be isolated.

By the use of the terms microcosm and macrocosm, I refer to socioeconomic conditions in which urban populations lived when mankind first felt that it was able to cope with city life. I refer to those crowded conditions when European populations lived behind city walls and to the squalor of the slums that must have existed there, the fleas, the lice, and the rats, and the great plagues that arose from these conditions (Zinsser 1935), as well as to the filth in the streets and the polluted water supplies. All these conditions are man made and are what we regard today as primitive sanitary conditions. And yet they are little worse than some of the ways of living, both urban and rural, that have grown up in the mid-twentieth century in our industrial civilization: the pollution of our atmosphere and our water courses, the incorrect use of pesticides, and countless other things. Attempts to improve conditions come under the heading of environmental sanitation, and urban (and rural) renewal—not to speak of our changing social and political philosophy.

These features, or at least some of them may concern medical students or the ordinary physician only from a general or moral point of view, whether they have epidemiological interests or not. Indeed, more appropriately, these matters belong in the fields of those who devote their energies to careers in public health than they do to those devoting their full energies to the practice of medicine. This recalls the ideals of the late C.-E. A. Winslow of Yale, who never tired of urging that public health departments should develop the social machinery to "ensure to every individual in the community a standard of living adequate for the maintenance of health" (Winslow 1920).

Winslow gave his definition of public health [2] in 1920 and it

[2] Public health is the science and the art of preventing disease, prolonging life, and promoting physical health and efficiency through organized community efforts for the sanitation of the environment, the control of community infections, the education of the individual in principles of personal hygiene, the organization of medical and nursing service for the early diagnosis and preventive treatment of disease, and the development of the social machinery which will ensure to every individual in the community a standard of living adequate for the maintenance of health.

9

has stood the test of time with few modifications. However, today the medical profession is as involved in the maintenance of public health as is the public health profession. It is, I believe, part of the doctor's job, or the clinical investigator's job, and certainly the clinical epidemiologist's job to be concerned about the intimate and even the public ways of living of communities, and their adequacy for the maintenance of health.

PRACTITIONERS OF EPIDEMIOLOGY

The health-department epidemiologist is a special kind of epidemiologist usually concerned with large populations and the biostatistical aspects of his science. He is in a position to practice epidemiology on a broad scale, dealing with large numbers and wide areas. His functions may include measurements of the effect of climate, usually within a given district, on the frequency of a disease such as pneumonia; or, as an urban epidemiologist, he may study local social conditions and their effects upon the prevalence of tuberculosis or ischemic heart disease. On the other hand, he may be concerned with the ecology of insect-borne diseases in rural areas, with nutritional deficiencies such as pellagra, with diabetes or obesity, with industrial disease, with the pollution of air or watercourses, or with accidents in the home or on the highways. Furthermore the therapeutic duties which his tasks entail take no small part of his time.

The clinical epidemiologist may have similar interests, but his is a more intimate task. He is to the statistical epidemiologist what a gardener is to a farmer. He can start with a single patient and his family, and branch out cautiously into the community. His first efforts are to search out and discover the presence of clinical or subclinical disease (clusters of disease) similar to that of his original patient. These may be associated with the patient's kindred, his locale, his occupation, ways of living, and so on—a true exercise in clinical investigation. I can find no better way of describing these activities than by turning to three British sources for a description of the work of academic clinical epidemiologists. One of these comes from J. N. Morris (1964) who has steadfastly emphasized that doctors have both much to learn from and much to contribute to epidemiology in helping to complete the clinical picture and the natural history of disease. Another is that of C. M. Fletcher (1963) who says, "If the work of clinicians and epidemiologists is indeed in continuity then it is essential that they should be in continuous professional contact." And another is that of Sir James Spence (1953), who says, "If clinical research is to be used to get the full picture of disease, it must equip itself to carry observations beyond hospitals. . . . The methodology of planned clinical observation . . . of the population will become a responsibility of medical schools. . . . If they fail, it is difficult to see how else it can be done."

Much more will be said in the following chapters about how doctors have changed. It would be unrealistic not to warn the reader about this. There is no question about our epidemiologically minded clinician being the exceptional physician or pediatrician; certainly he is not the rank and file engaged in the practice of medicine. On the average at least, the modern practice of medicine apparently depends on only a rare home visit. According to a recent *Medical Economics* survey, quoted by Dickinson Richards (1965), even the general practitioner confines almost his entire working time to intramural practice, with an average of 126 office visits, 16 hospital calls, and only 5 house visits a week. How can the intimate practice of medicine survive on any such program? The pendulum will swing no doubt, not only in the way of providing adequate and intimate medical services but also for the physician's return to the fulfillment of the ideals of Sir James Spence.

BIBLIOGRAPHY

Blakiston's New Gould Medical Dictionary, 1949. Philadelphia: Blakiston Co.

BURNET, F. M. 1940. *Biological aspects of infectious disease.* New York: Macmillan Co.

BURNET, SIR MACFARLANE. 1953. *The natural history of infectious disease.* 2d ed. London: Cambridge University Press.

FLETCHER, C. M. 1963. Epidemiologist and clinical investigator. *Proc. Roy. Soc. Med. (Sect. Epidemiol. and Prev. Med.)* **56**:851–58.

FROST, W. H. 1928a. Epidemiology. In *Nelson's loose-leaf living medicine*. New York: Thos. Nelson & Sons. Also in *Papers of Wade Hampton Frost M. D.*, ed. K. F. MAXCY. 1941. New York: Oxford University Press.

GORDON, J. E. 1955. Population pathology. *Trans. Coll. Phys.* (*Phila.*) **23**:1.

GREENWOOD, M. 1939. Preface. In *Epidemiology in country practice*. W. N. PICKLES. Baltimore: Williams and Wilkins Co.

KRUTCH, J. W. 1964. On being an amateur naturalist and Man's ancient powerful link to nature. In: *If you don't mind my saying so. Essays on Man and Nature*, pp. 331–48. New York: Wm. Sloane.

LEAVELL, H. R. and CLARK, E. G. 1958. *Preventive medicine for the doctor in his community. An epidemiologic approach.* New York: McGraw-Hill Book Co.

MORRIS, J. N. 1964. *Uses of epidemiology.* 2d ed. Edinburgh: E. & S. Livingstone.

NICOLLE, C. 1939. *Destin des maladies infecteuses.* 3d ed. Paris: Presses Universitaires de France.

PAUL, J. R. 1938. Clinical epidemiology. *J. Clin. Investigation* **17**: 539–41.

RICHARDS, D. W. 1965. The hospital and the city. *Pharos.* **28**:35–38.

ROUS, P. 1938. Nature and the doctor. *Science*, **88**:483.

RYLE, J. A. 1948a. *The natural history of disease.* 2d ed. p. 446. London: Oxford University Press.

———. 1948b. *Changing disciplines: Lectures on the history, method and motives of social pathology.* London: Oxford University Press.

———. 1949. Social Pathology. In *Social medicine, its derivatives and objectives,* I. GALDSTON (ed.). New York: Commonwealth Fund.

SIGERIST, H. S. 1946. *The University at the Crossroads.* New York: H. Shuman.

SPENCE, J. 1950. Family studies in preventive medicine. *New Engl. J. Med.* **243**:205.

SMITH, T. 1934. *Parasitism and disease.* Princeton: Princeton University Press.

Webster's New World Dictionary of the American Language. 1957. Cleveland: World Publishing Co.

WELCH, W. H. 1916. Institute of Hygiene. In Rockefeller Foundation Annual Report, pp. 415–27. New York.

WINSLOW, C.-E. A. 1920. The untilled fields of Public Health. *Science* **51** (No. 1306): 21–33.

ZINSSER, H. 1935. *Rats, lice and history.* Boston: Little, Brown & Co.

———. 1940. *As I remember him.* Boston: Little, Brown & Co.

CHAPTER II

History—From Ancient Greece
to 1800

Man's efforts to find out about disease, plague, and pestilence are probably as old as his efforts to create a religion for himself. When one considers the devastating epidemics which swept the known world in Greek and Roman times and during the Middle Ages, it seems probable that almost all thinking people became epidemiologists to some extent. It is also fair to say that a few of their explanations about man's responsibility for epidemics were not so wide of the mark as some historians have insisted. Even today man-made disease is commoner than many people may care to admit.

The evil work of demons, God's wrath, and God's plans regarding the manner in which man was to live, were the usual explanations for epidemic disease in the early stages of what we may call civilization; these attitudes have been well described by my senior colleague, the late C.-E. A. Winslow in his books dealing with the evolution of ideas that led to the control of certain epidemic diseases (1934, 1943, 1952). The transition from supernatural to natural explanations of disease may be said to mark the beginnings of modern epidemiology. This took place, according to Major Greenwood (1921), "like almost everything that makes life worth living, in ancient Greece."

Hippocrates, in his discourses on "Airs, Waters, and Places," indicated his respect for elements in the environment as a direct or contributing cause to many different types of illness and their effect on the peoples living under different climatic conditions. Among sayings attributed to him is the following remark: "such affections are divine, and so are all others, no one being more divine than any other; all are alike and all divine. Each of them has a nature of its own, and no one arises without a natural cause." (Adams trans., 1886, I, p. 178).

This ancient example of observation and reason could have become the basis of an inductive method of studying the behavior of disease. Had it been followed by others who came after Hippocrates, it might have advanced man's comprehension of disease by many centuries. There also seems to be a respect, in the works of Hippocrates, for what might be called a balance between God and nature, which might still profitably apply to our thinking about this subject.

To appreciate what the thinking must have been during the long period of more than two thousand years, extending from the time of Hippocrates to that of Pasteur, one might try to visualize what epidemics meant in that period—their frequency and their magnitude. Indeed, we need go no farther back than the late eighteenth and early nineteenth centuries to find the European world and colonial America still plagued with a variety of epidemic diseases, the causes of which were almost wholly mysterious as well as frightening to physicians and laymen alike. Fear and ignorance prevailed right up to the last third of the nineteenth century, until the inception of the concept of microbes as causes of infectious diseases—even the twentieth century had its share of terror.[1]

As long as man lived a nomadic life in small and scattered communities, he was in less danger from devastating epidemics of infectious disease than after he began to develop agriculture, to form larger communities, and to live a more sedentary existence. When the element of crowding came into play, that is, when larger numbers of people than had hitherto existed were crowded together, the habits and ways of living which had been adequate for nomadic life were found to be inadequate for village life. There was an increased likelihood not only that an

---

[1] The pandemic of influenza of 1918–19, whose viral cause was unknown at the time, might be said to have struck just as much fear into the souls of men as the great plagues of the eighteenth century.

infection would spread but that the infecting agent (or parasite) would persist within the community for longer periods of time. At least this is the way one views the situation from the present vantage point. Epidemiological principles were probably the same, although theoretically the actual viruses, bacteria, or poisons that afflicted mankind two thousand years ago may have been different from those with which we are most familiar today, and the diseases may therefore have been different. Within the past forty years "new" infectious diseases have been recognized, many of which seem never to have been described before. Some of these, like *encephalitis lethargica,* apparently have come and gone. Many an industrial disease, such as benzol poisoning or carbon tetrachloride poisoning, could not have existed several centuries ago. The rapid rise in incidence of carcinoma of the lung is another modern phenomenon.

One of the worst afflictions that beset mankind over many centuries was bubonic plague, a disease which is usually spread through the agency of the rat flea, although its most severe form, pneumonic plague, is transmitted from person to person by so-called direct transmission. In cities, particularly in crowded cities where rats abounded, conditions must have been ideal for the spread of this infection, especially since the population was unaware of the nature of the disease, its animal reservoir, or the arthropod vector. An early epidemic was the Great Plague of Justinian which began in the East in A.D. 532 and circled the Mediterranean in four long periods of about fifteen years each. With its ultimate departure, originally populous countries "were left like deserts." The Black Death of the Middle Ages, so called because in those serious and fatal cases in which the lungs were frequently affected, the difficulty in breathing and resulting cyanosis gave rise to a bluish or purplish color of the face and lips, was probably a severe type of this same disease. To say that the mortality from the plague from 1350 to 1700 was extensive is an understatement, for it is estimated that during its waves of greatest prevalence there were times when one quarter of the population of Europe died (Nohl 1924, Smith 1943). There was agreement that the origin of plague was in the Far East, probably in China, but there was no inkling regarding the cause and nature of this disease, which affected rich and poor alike. A usual interpretation was that it represented the visitation of an angry God upon a sinful people, an explanation that was as good as any at the time and not so wide of the mark when one imagines the unsanitary conditions which must have prevailed throughout the crowded primitive cities—the character of the water supply, the filth in the streets, the rats, and the lice. Apparently it has taken man many centuries to learn to live an urban existence, and he probably still has much to learn (Zinsser 1935).

How many infectious diseases, either epidemic or endemic, took their toll among non-immune or semi-immune populations throughout the past six or seven hundred years is hard to estimate: smallpox, measles, scarlet fever, and diphtheria are a few which are known to have existed. Cholera was probably responsible for a major share of the deaths. Sydenham described it in Britain in 1669. India had long been its home; its forays into foreign lands probably became more frequent after that country was opened up to trade and travel by the East India Company. In this connection it is easy to appreciate the development of the concept that pestilence came from abroad—the plague from China, cholera from India. Similarly, when syphilis was first recognized after the supposed siege of Naples, it was called "the French disease." Four hundred years later, in 1918, pandemic influenza was described during the early days of its appearance, as the "Spanish" influenza. This placing of the blame for pestilence upon one's neighbors had considerable basis in fact. Often a whole community existed happily for years without a given infection, and then with the advent of visitors came the introduction of a new infectious agent. A modern example might be tuberculosis or poliomyelitis among Eskimos; with the introduction of these diseases devastating results ensued. Blaming one's neighbors or visitors for pestilence was also sometimes an escape from the embarrassment of having to admit that the epidemic flourished because of one's own local "bad habits."

Classical examples of devastation wrought by epidemics were

those in colonial America. With the introduction of smallpox and measles virus into the non-immune native population of North American Indians, some of these tribes were all but wiped out. The isolated position of the colonists also allowed many to grow up without childhood infection by measles virus, so that adult colonists suffered terribly from this disease when it was introduced periodically. Such introductions of the virus were few and far between. In other words measles died out between epidemics in colonial America, resulting in severe epidemics when reintroduced occasionally from without. Since the infectious period of a case of measles is short, and the length of its incubation period is about two weeks, it is not remarkable that the virus did not often get to America from Europe until the voyage across the Atlantic became shorter than a month. Indeed, for a long time, conditions necessitated the development not of secondary but of tertiary cases on shipboard, if a person were to reach America in the infectious stage. Not until communities or groups of communities became large enough to maintain the measles virus during interepidemic periods did the adult population become almost wholly immune to measles, as in most modern urban communities.

Other terrible scourges in colonial America were diphtheria and yellow fever. For reasons that are not clear today, the former was a disease of epidemic potentialities which carried with it a higher mortality in the seventeenth and early eighteenth centuries than it did in the nineteenth century. Yellow fever was another fearful pestilence which swept the colonies in extensive waves according to the earliest records. Although yellow fever was established more or less endemically in the islands of the West Indies, in Mexico, and on the South American continent, urban epidemics broke out from time to time in the coastal seaports of the United States. The onset of such an epidemic was usually during the summer and coincided with the arrival of a ship from the West Indies. In the eighteenth century the epidemics of yellow fever in Philadelphia alone, notably those of 1793 and the years immediately following, were responsible for more than ten thousand deaths. The controversies that raged among local physicians and laymen over what was responsible for these terrible visitations were as bitter as any that might rage between a group of ministers arguing a point of religious dogma (Rush 1794, Corner 1948). Was it contagious? Was it due to a polluted atmosphere or to rotting coffee? It was not until a hundred years later that the first answer to this puzzle was given when Carlos Finlay, a physician in Havana, advised Walter Reed, an American army surgeon, about experiments that led to the recognition of the mosquito's role in the transmission of yellow fever. This in turn led to the discovery, a generation later in West Africa, of the causative virus and subsequently to the development of an effective vaccine. Still later it was found that monkeys represented an important animal reservoir of the virus. And the story is not yet finished.

It is easy to imagine the intense curiosity and the vital interest of physicians and laymen—indeed the gulf between them was probably not great—when it came to explaining or dealing with epidemic disease. Not only were the causes wholly mysterious, but the public was willing to try almost anything when it came to devising programs of treatment for the sick and programs for the prevention of disease. Into this field of speculation, theorists and observers flocked during the seventeenth, eighteenth, and most of the nineteenth centuries, and there is little reason to believe that the speculations of the doctors were much better than those of laymen. Dominant was the idea that environmental disturbances, whether of meteorologic or geologic origin, acted as precipitating causes of epidemics. This probably had some basis in fact; if the water supply to a village or city was disrupted by an earthquake, typhoid, cholera, or dysentery might have followed or increased in the wake of the accident. Thus, an intimate association in the minds of these early "epidemiologists" between the earthquake and the pestilence would be understandable.

What one should remember here is that although they had a fair concept of contagion, the great majority of those who pondered over the causes of epidemic disease had little or no idea of *contagium vivum,* or a microbial cause for a disease. How could one have studied epidemiology in the seventeenth century

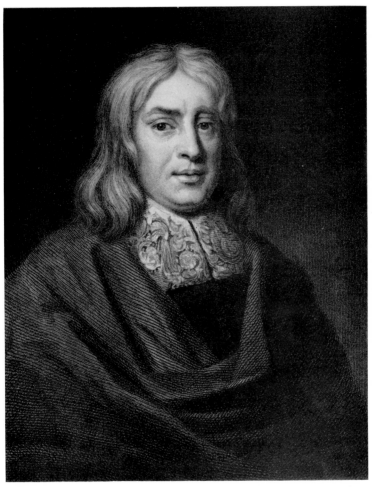

FIG. 1. Thomas Sydenham (1624–89). Engraving by E. Scriven from the portrait at All Soul's College, Oxford, painted by John Jackson, R.A. (1778–1831). (Reproduced by courtesy of the Yale University Medical Library.)

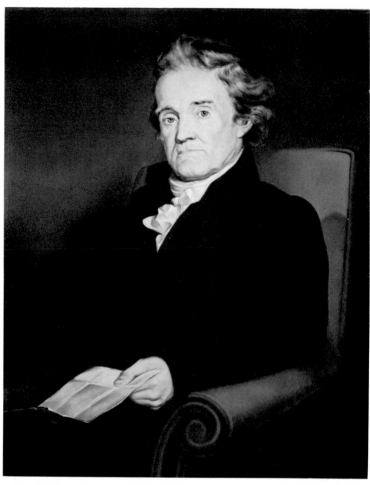

Fig. 2. Noah Webster (1758–1843). Copy of a portrait by P. F and R. F. Zallinger from the original by Samuel F. B. Morse. (Reproduced by courtesy of the Yale University Art Gallery.)

except by concerning oneself with the two major extra-microbial factors, host resistance and the environment? As there was scant knowledge of the host and his immunity, it was natural to turn to the environment; consequently, environmental epidemiology held sway.

Another difficulty confronting epidemiologists of the period was that the diseases of which they spoke had little individuality. Many diseases were so poorly defined that only when they appeared in epidemic form did their character come to the fore. Not until the end of the eighteenth century did infectious diseases emerge as individual entities from a jumble of fevers— fevers both short and long in duration, some remittent and others intermittent, some with spots on the skin and some without.

Only a few personalities from this period will be singled out for discussion as outstanding figures in the history of ideas about the causation of various diseases. One controversial figure was Thomas Sydenham (1624–89) of London, sometimes known as the father of epidemiology, who can be said to have at least started a new trend in epidemiological thinking. Coming from a background dominated by the speculations of the iatrochemists, he stressed clinical observation, reviving, after some two thousand years, the Hippocratic method of recording accounts of various cases. This called for descriptions of disease and their characteristic lesions at the bedside and at the autopsy table. Against considerable opposition Sydenham proposed that the individuality of some diseases was sufficiently plain to allow them to be classified, as botanists had done in their description of plants.

It may be hard for us to follow his thinking about the individuality of different diseases. He believed in their individuality only up to a certain point. His ideas were based on what he called epidemic constitutions, or seasons, which might last for several years within a population, such as that of London, which for that season underwent its own special fevers, agues, plagues, and pestilences. It appeared that an "epidemic constitution was characterized by a sequence of related diseases and that a particular disease was strictly specific within this constitutional framework (Sydenham 1717; see Riesman 1927 for bibliography of Sydenham's works). The development of this idea was carried forward after Sydenham's death by Francois Boissier de Sauvages in France, who, as a botanist-physician and as a friend and correspondent of Linnaeus in Sweden, sought to group diseases in classes, orders, and genera. This idea of creating classes and orders of diseases at a time when so little was known about them may have been as tentative as attempts are to classify viruses today, but it furthered the concept that if one could impart individuality to certain diseases, their characteristic behavior could next be considered (Sauvages 1731). Actually this early concept led directly to the current system of disease nomenclature, on which modern medicine leans heavily. The classification by Sauvages was a forerunner of many such classifications, or nosologies. Their history was well reviewed a generation ago in a small but important book by Knud Faber (1923) of Denmark.

Another figure among the many who emerged in the eighteenth century was Noah Webster (1758–1843), the New England lexicographer. He was not a physician but was fascinated by the idea of pestilence and spent an immense amount of time collecting information about epidemics, speculating on their genesis and course, and recording local views. He was a strong disbeliever in the idea of infection; for him it was the climate that usually was at fault. Like a number of his predecessors he had special theories about causal relationships between disease and earthquakes, volcanic eruptions, and other spectacular phenomena (Webster 1799). He claimed that his creed was "As facts are the basis of human knowledge, it is of great importance to collect them," but he seems to have been more devoted to his own opinions, many of which he had reached, as a good lexicographer should, in his library. In any event he was the first American epidemiologist. Although many of his conclusions were apparently based on folklore, hearsay, and tall stories, much of his epidemiological lore is as acceptable today as the pompous explanations about epidemic disease that doctors of medicine put forth in the years immediately following him (Winslow 1934).

Some of Websters notions about infectivity hark back to

Sydenham. He was much concerned with a fundamental epidemiologic question many must have pondered: Were *people* infected and infective, or was the whole *place* infective? As arguments swung in the latter direction, one can easily imagine how the concept of a deadly miasma and the pollution of the atmosphere came in. The failure to realize at that time that a polluted water supply could give rise to typhoid fever or that a mosquito could carry the yellow fever virus are but two examples that point up the difficulties of trying to solve these questions in a library. Thus Webster conceived of the infective influence as a chemical gaseous agent (septic acid) which operated at a maximum range of perhaps ten paces. This could affect animals and birds as well as human beings. He quotes Lind's description of an epidemic occuring in Bethlehem, Connecticut, in 1760:

In November the town of Bethlehem was assailed by an inflammatory fever, with symptoms of typhus, which in the course of the following winter carried off about 40 of the inhabitants. . . . During the epidemic, a flock of quails flew over the chimney of a house in which were several diseased persons and five of them fell dead on the spot.

BIBLIOGRAPHY

ADAMS, FRANCIS (trans.). 1886. *The genuine works of Hippocrates.* New York: Wm. Wood & Co.

CAULFIELD, E. 1939. The throat distemper. *Yale Jour. Biol. Med. Suppl.*

CORNER, G. W. 1948. *The autobiography of Benjamin Rush.* Princeton: Princeton University Press.

DUFFY, J. 1953. *Epidemics in colonial America.* Baton Rouge: Louisiana State University Press.

FABER, K. 1923. *Nosography.* New York: Paul B. Hoeber.

GREENHILL, W. A. 1848. Translation of RHAZES' *Treatise on the smallpox and measles.* London: New Sydenham Society.

GREENWOOD, M. 1921. History of Medicine. *Proc. Roy. Soc. Med.,* **14**:3.

——. 1932. *Epidemiology—historical and experimental.* Baltimore: Johns Hopkins Press.

NOHL, J. 1924. *The Black Death: A chronicle of the plague.* Translated by C. H. CLARKE. New York: Harper & Bros.

PECHEY, JOHN. 1717. *The whole works* of THOMAS SYDENHAM, translated from the original Latin. 7th ed. London: M. Wellington.

RIESMAN, D. 1926. *Thos. Sydenham, clinician.* New York: Paul B. Hoeber. Includes bibliography of Sydenham's works.

RUSH, BENJAMIN. 1794. *An account of the bilious remitting yellow fever as it appeared in the city of Philadelphia in the year 1793.* 2d ed. Philadelphia: Thos. Dobson.

SAUVAGES, F. B. DE. 1731. *Traité des classes des maladies.* Montpellier.

SMITH, G. 1943. *Plague on us.* New York: Commonwealth Fund.

VIETS, H. R. 1949. George Cheyne, 1673–1743. *Bull. Hist. Med.* **23:** 435–52.

WEBSTER, NOAH. 1799. *A brief history of epidemic and pestilential diseases; with the principal phenomena of the physical world which precede and accompany them.* Hartford: Hudson & Goodwin.

WINSLOW, C.-E. A. 1934. The epidemiology of Noah Webster. *Conn. Acad. Arts and Sciences,* **32:**21–109.

———. 1943. *The conquest of epidemic disease.* Princeton: Princeton University Press.

———. 1952. *The history of American epidemiology,* chap. 1. St. Louis: C. V. Mosby Co.

CHAPTER III

History—The Nineteenth Century and the Beginning of the Modern Period

Early in the nineteenth century a number of significant clinical and epidemiological observations were made that paved the way for the identification of individual diseases and for an appreciation of their specific epidemiologic behavior. Measles and smallpox had long been identified and documented epidemiologically, but the fevers, whether short, intermittent, or "continued," were in a confused state. A good example of clinical epidemiology in early America can be found in the observations of Nathan Smith (1762–1829) on typhoid fever (1824). In the course of his extensive practice in New England he came to know this disease, which was then called typhous fever (Paul, 1930). This disease had enough individuality to deserve a name of its own, although previously it had not been singled out from the other "continued" fevers. A continued fever consisted of any fever for which there was no obvious cause and which lasted more than a week. This must have included a hodgepodge of diseases. Out of this jumble Nathan Smith identified typhoid fever, from both its clinical and epidemiological behavior, noting particularly its comings and goings in small New England villages and its capacity to immunize. As a result of these observations, he came to regard this disease as a definite entity. Upon this point—the individuality of typhoid fever, Smith's views were original and understandably at odds with contemporary medical doctrines. In a book review in the *New England Journal of Medicine* in 1824 which was critical of his *Practical Essay on Typhous Fever,* we find the following contemporary expression of skepticism:

> Dr. Smith says that typhus is a distinct disease, a disease *sui generis,* a specific disease, and *not a state of fever,* plainly implying, if words can imply anything plainly, that he does not view typhus as a fever in the common sense of the word. Now that there can be a strictly specific disease thus merging itself in an affection arising from ordinary causes, is contrary to all analogy and experience; we do not find it true of any disease allowedly specific and we are not yet prepared to believe it.

Seventy-five years later Dr. W. H. Welch (1901–2) was to liken Nathan Smith's essay to "a fresh breeze from the sea amid the dreary and stifling writings of most of his contemporaries."

America's next contribution to the history of typhoid fever is well known. In 1834 William Gerhard, a young American physician who had worked with Louis in Paris, returned to Philadelphia to assume the position of resident physician at the Pennsylvania Hospital. Here he found that the cases of continued fever then prevalent, were identical, clinically and anatomically, with the typhoid fever which Louis had found to be characterized by intestinal lesions. About two years later when an epidemic of what we now call typhus developed in Philadelphia, Gerhard was able to differentiate this disease, which he had seen in Edinburgh, from typhoid fever (Gerhard 1837). It was thus established that the two diseases, typhoid fever (subsequently shown to be spread by contaminated water or food or human contact) and typhus (shown still later to be spread by the body louse or rat flea) were two "continued fevers" with individual characteristics. This was a development which called first, for the *identification* of the two diseases, so that their individual behavior and epidemiology could be considered and, secondly, for some therapeutic application of these observations.

After 1800 medicine moved faster toward a scientific approach to disease. During this time there was constant groping for an understanding of the causes of and classification of diseases, particularly of fevers. Not recognizing such causes as microbes or parasites, the investigator or physician naturally sought an explanation in the environment. Today it is not always easy to differentiate outbreaks of infectious (contagious) diseases from outbreaks of non-infectious diseases; how much more difficult it must have been half a century before the days of Pasteur. This must have been particularly confusing in the case of "epidemics" of non-infectious disease such as eighteenth-century lead colic, both in England and this country. Some of these lead poisoning cases were caused by drinking cider or distilled liquor that had been in contact with lead pipes or lead containers. A much more recent example is that of pellagra, where aggregates of cases in certain parts of the United States suggested for a while that this disease was an infectious condition. Only as a result of certain astute observations was it found that local kinds of diets were responsible for pellagra.

Another milestone in epidemiological thinking was reached one hundred years ago, in the pre-bacterial era, with the recognition that an infectious disease could be spread through the agency of contaminated drinking water. This discovery singled out an undesirable and correctable feature within the environment. Thus John Snow's observations on the Broad Street pump in London as a source of contaminated water responsible for the spread of cholera in 1854 was a revolutionary landmark in the history of enteric disease and environmental sanitation, of which more will be mentioned later (see Snow 1936).

William Budd of Bristol, England, studying another enteric disease—typhoid fever—reached the same conclusion five years later in 1859, that Snow had reached with cholera (Budd 1873). Here again the observations on the epidemiologic significance of the pollution of water supply were not completely new. That the drinking of bad water can lead to illness is an age-old concept; but that Snow was able to point to the exact source of contamination, charting the distribution of cholera cases among those who drank water from a certain well, not only established a principle but at the same time indicated that something might be done about the situation. Epidemiologists have singled out the water-borne, or enteric, diseases as a special family of preventable diseases ever since.

By 1850 scientific medicine was on the march. First had come the French school with Laennec, Louis, and Brettoneau, then the rise of the German school with Virchow, Cohnheim, Koch, and a host of others. But it was the era of Pasteur, from 1860 to 1890,

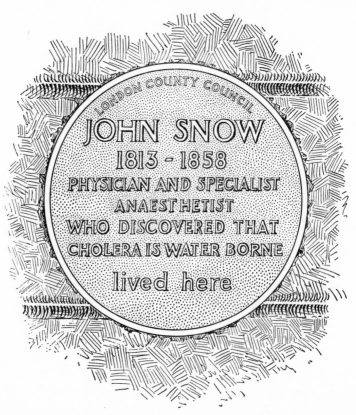

FIG. 3. This plaque, which has been placed on John Snow's house in Sackville Street, London, as a reminder of his contribution to epidemiology and to the public health, speaks for itself. It is perhaps a more modest monument than many others erected to individuals whose contributions to humanity have not been as great. (Sketched from a photograph kindly supplied by Dr. Ian Taylor, London County Council.)

that brought the germ theory of infectious disease into being. The whole concept of the cause of infections was thus revolutionized, with great emphasis placed on bacteria (or at least on microbes) as *the* cause of such diseases. The credit cannot be wholly ascribed to Pasteur for this revolution, as its seeds had been sown (in a poor climate and on rocky soil) some two hundred years before; and in the nineteenth century, just before Pasteur's time, the idea that certain skin "infections" could be caused by tiny parasites, smaller than the itch mite, was recognized. Furthermore, the experience in Europe and America with inoculation for smallpox, and later with Jenner's cowpox in which the "lymph" harbored an infectious agent, had already covered more than a hundred years. But it was the introduction by Pasteur in France and by Koch in Germany of evidence of the existence of microbes as infectious agents and the development of methods of handling these agents that brought forth a whole new concept—the science of infectious disease.

Many have claimed that Pasteur failed to recognize the importance of the susceptible or unsusceptible host because he was so preoccupied with the pathogenic organism. This is probably incorrect. Pasteur's immediate followers were the ones who seemed to have overemphasized the microbe or, epidemiologically speaking, the seed. Pasteur himself did an immense amount of work on induced immunity, and it is alleged that at the end of his life he said, "Le microbe n'est rien, le terrain est tout" (Selye 1955). In any event, the spirit of the first fifty years of the bacteriological era was so to emphasize the role of parasites in inducing disease that for the time being the host (the soil) and the epidemiologic climate received much less attention. This is understandable enough when one considers the excitement that must have gone along with the new methods being devised for growing and testing the properties of bacteria, methods that had a special appeal to scientists. Something barely comprehended before could now be seen and measured. On the other hand, human resistance and the role of the environment in the transmission or the maintenance of infectious disease did not lend themselves so readily to accurate measurements and accordingly were neglected.

One of the sometimes forgotten nineteenth-century champions of the epidemiological climate was Professor Max von Pettenkofer (1819–1901) of Munich. He was an early proponent of the concept that multiple factors were at play in the causation and spread of infectious disease. His ability to define these other factors was so limited that he did not get far, but he had a clear vision that one of the necessary conditions for the spread of certain infections was a susceptible population (Hume 1927).

Although Pettenkofer lived to see the birth of the germ theory and the great advances made by the science of bacteriology in the 1880's he was not swept along by this movement; he never even accepted the idea that infection was conveyed by bacteria. So opposed was he that he is said to have swallowed a culture of cholera vibrios to prove their harmlessness. Indeed he seems to have expended more energy in belittling the germ theory than in building his concepts of measuring the role of the environment. His theories on the cause of epidemics have in large measure been discarded, but he must be given credit for recognizing that the pathogenesis of enteric disease went beyond the germ theory. It was not so simple a process as others after him claimed. History has amply confirmed this fact (Galdston 1954).

Another nineteenth-century figure who deserves a place in the history of epidemiology was Peter Ludwig Panum, a Danish physician who described the extraordinarily severe epidemic of measles which occurred in 1846 in the non-immune adult and juvenile population of the remote Faroe Islands (Panum 1846). It was an example of a common disease behaving differently in two different populations, one (semi-immune) in Denmark and the other (non-immune) on a remote island. Because this virus infection is a mild disease in children from four to fifteen years of age, and because most cases of measles today in an urban population are in that age group, measles is usually called a mild children's disease. Its ability to confer immunity on the once-infected individual leaves the usual adult population of most cities protected for life. But where childhood measles has failed to occur, a person can reach the age of thirty years and still be non-immune. The infection, if acquired after childhood, can be very severe, so that in a population of adult non-immunes, measles can become a devastating plague; this is often true when the virus is introduced into isolated parts of the world.

Panum's observation, calling attention as it did to the importance of the immune status of the population, was neither new nor unique, but it was dramatic enough to drive home a point of great epidemiologic significance.

The observations mentioned thus far were largely made by a few doctors who seemed to have been a little more curious than their fellows about the natural history of diseases. Their approach was that of dealing with cases of illness in individual patients or groups of patients and with the impact of these cases upon the welfare of the community only in a general sort of way. But it presently became clear that if the mode of spread of a given disease and its pathogenesis were to be unraveled, more was needed than mere observations on patients coupled with some general knowledge of the community. The development of our subject depended not only upon careful diagnosis and astute clinical observations but also on other types of information which might concern both sick and well members of the family or of the local community. Today this includes a definition of the size of a given community and its geographical limits; it includes also much detailed information about the character of the population involved and the distribution of various racial, socioeconomic, and age groups as they exist at a given period of time. But most of all it calls for an orderly arrangement of these facts into chains of inference extending beyond the bounds of direct observation.

The development of this point of view demands some elementary comprehension of and respect for statistics and some knowledge of population data, demography so-called. Clinicians have long had the reputation of disregarding statistics, and it is easy for those who have had little or no biostatistical training to err in their estimates of a given community situation, especially in determining whether a given condition is frequent or rare.[1]

[1] Although the argument that clinicians should treat every case individually still holds, physicians more and more are using methods which require statistical treatment. Concerning this Dr. Warren Weaver (1960), President of the Alfred P. Sloan Foundation and former Director for Medical Sciences of the Rockefeller Foundation, wrote: "The automatic discarding of evidence because it is statistical is unscientific and wholly unwarranted. Statistical evidence is, in essentially non-trivial cases, the only sort of evidence we can possibly have."

Consequently it was the introduction of a discriminating attitude toward statistics that was in part responsible for developing the field of epidemiology as a science in its own right and put an end to the era when conclusions were drawn and generalizations put forth based only on clinical impressions unaccompanied by demographic measurements.

Actually the statistical science of epidemiology may be said to have been born and raised as a neglected child in the late seventeenth century in England. It got its impetus almost wholly from the tabulations of vital statistics collected by a man named John Graunt (1620–74). According to Greenwood (1948), Graunt was not only the first to measure the difference between urban and rural mortality and to devise methods of estimating populations by sampling; he was the first constructive critic of medical statistical data. Later, and again in England, the value of these measurements was reappraised in connection with Farr's application of mathematics to vital statistics. Thus a means of furnishing the first adequate description of morbidity and mortality rates was demonstrated. The significance of developments in this field needs little comment or description here (Greenwood 1948).

In the United States, one who early realized the worth of morbidity statistics was Dr. C. V. Chapin. As city registrar of Providence, Rhode Island, from 1888 until 1932, he succeeded in making the registration reports of that city models of accuracy and completeness. His work was an example of the careful recording of data over a considerable number of years by an individual intent upon determining the behavior of certain diseases within the community he served and apparently knew as well as a country pastor knows his flock. Statistical epidemiologists have subsequently used Chapin's data to considerable advantage, and a generation of students of biostatistics have been brought up on them (Wilson et al. 1939; Cassedy 1962).

Later W. H. Frost (1928, p. 163) did much to transform epidemiology in the United States from a loose discipline to an analytical and productive science. Frost's work began with careful clinical observations, many of which were made as part of a series of field observations; this was followed up with population measurements. Then with orderly precision the data were subjected to biostatistical treatment. It had taken almost four thousand years for epidemiology to emerge as a discipline ready, by about 1920, to stand on its own feet among the medical arts and sciences. To Frost also we owe in part the concept that an epidemic is but a temporary phase in the occurrence of any disease and as such epidemiology represented more than the study of epidemics and was a science ready to be applied to all diseases.

This brings us back to present-day developments and definitions, reminding us that epidemiology is essentially a technique by which the many circumstances under which disease (any disease) occurs may be measured. This modern concept of epidemiology came into being in a number of different places more or less simultaneously when the background finally became ripe for such a development. It was also at about the time that the medical profession began to realize what immense possibilities there were in clinical investigation in epidemiologic fields. This represented a development which took place in the early 1920's, and has been described, as far as infectious disease is concerned, as the next step beyond bacteriology. It grew out of a need to search for causes of disease that were not limited to the etiologic agent which directly initiates the process—causes, some of which the hospital or public health laboratory could elucidate, some they could not. Up to this point, or at least during the previous two generations, as Gordon has pointed out (1952), bacteriology and the epidemiology of infectious diseases had almost appeared to be one and the same science. Now the conviction arose that "bacteriology was *not* epidemiology," for the latter goes far beyond the petrie dish, far beyond the test tube. As a matter of fact it had gone far beyond the idea that a single etiologic agent was responsible for most disease. The ferreting out of multiple causes had become a science in itself.

BIBLIOGRAPHY

Budd, W. 1873. *Typhoid fever; its nature, mode of spreading and prevention.* London: Longmans, Green & Co.

CASSEDY, J. H. 1962. *Charles V. Chapin and the Public Health Movement*. Cambridge: Harvard University Press.

FROST, W. H. 1928. Epidemiology. In *Nelson's loose-leaf living medicine*. II. New York: Thos. Nelson & Sons.

GALDSTON, I. (ed.). 1954. *Beyond the germ theory*. New York: Health Education Council, New York Academy of Medicine.

GERHARD, W. W. 1837. On the typhus fever which occurred at Philadelphia in the spring and summer of 1836. *Am. J. Med. Sci.* **40**:25.

GORDON, J. E. 1952. The twentieth century—yesterday, today and tomorrow. In *The history of American epidemiology*. St. Louis: C. V. Mosby Co.

GREENWOOD, M. 1948. *Some British pioneers of social medicine*. London: Oxford University Press.

HUME, E. E. 1927. *Max von Pettenkofer*. New York: Paul B. Hoeber.

PANAM, P. L. 1846. Observations made during the epidemic of measles on the Faroe Islands in the year 1846. Translated by the DELTA OMEGA SOCIETY. New York: American Public Health Association.

PAUL, J. R. 1930. Nathan Smith and typhoid fever. *Yale J. Biol. Med.* **2**:169.

SELYE, H. 1955. Stress and disease. *Science* **122**:625.

SMITH, N. 1824. *A practical essay on typhous fever*. New York: E. Bless & E. White.

SNOW, J. 1936. *Snow on cholera; being a reprint of two papers by John Snow, M.D.* Edited and with a biographical memoir by E. W. RICHARDSON; introduction by W. H. FROST. New York: Commonwealth Fund.

WEAVER, W. 1960. The disparagement of statistical evidence. *Science* **123**:1859.

WELCH, W. H. 1901. Relation of Yale to medicine. *Yale Med. J.* **8**:127.

WILSON, E. B., BENNETT, C., ALLEN, M., and WORCESTER, J. 1939. Measles and scarlet fever in Providence, R.I., 1929–1934, with respect to age and size of family. *Proc. Am. Phil. Soc.* **80**:357.

CHAPTER IV

Clinical Approaches to the Use of Epidemiology

As has already been suggested in a previous chapter, clinicians deal not only with patients, with their symptoms and lesions, but with the settings in which their troubles have arisen. How physicians get this information is not exactly our concern, but it is important that they get it if the clinical picture is to be complete. To attest is the modern fact that few textbooks of medicine today describe a noteworthy medical disease without a section on its epidemiology. Unlike the time-honored basic sciences or specialties of medicine that have pursued an analytical evolution, the epidemiologist has had to assume a more general point of view taking in the whole person, his family, and his surroundings. The specialist is concerned with a method, an anatomical tract, or an organ perhaps. He is careful to look at that aspect of an illness he knows best, necessarily limiting himself to treat his own specialty adequately. And this is a thoroughly valid approach that should not be allowed to suffer. But to offset the calamity of a patient or a family being split in too many "clinical" pieces, the epidemiologist is in a position to gather up the whole. If ever the doctrine of holism (Smuts 1926) could apply to medicine, it should apply to epidemiology.

Physicians have tried to be epidemiologists of one sort or another for a good many centuries, as the last chapters testify, but only recently have they begun to collect exact epidemiological measurements in the laboratory or elsewhere and to apply statistical methods to determine their significance. This has made all the difference in a discipline originally regarded from a purely observational standpoint.

The idea of relating disease prevalence to community conditions is certainly not new. The reports of the St. Andrew's Institute for Clinical Research (MacKenzie 1922–26) were perhaps an earlier expression of this same idea conceived in Scotland for clinicians by a clinician. Carrying this idea forward has been the undertaking of certain hospitals or clinics that have tried to establish an epidemiological tie-in with the medical practice of the community. A few of these are the medical organization in England in New Castle-upon-Tyne (Spence *et al.* 1950, 1954); and in the United States, in Cooperstown, N.Y. (Bordley 1950), and in Hunterdon, N.J. (Trussell 1955).

There also have been many sickness surveys carried out largely by research groups, the results of which will hardly be our concern. To set up such a program requires a certain supply of unrestricted funds and a team of skilled persons, requirements that may put such programs beyond the range of most physicians. Examples of such extensive surveys include the cardiac program in Framingham, Mass., and innumerable other surveys on cardiovascular disease in this country or abroad, either in industrial groups or communities; also the Community Health Study that has been undertaken at the Eastern Health District of Baltimore, Md., by the Johns Hopkins School of Hygiene (Downes 1950, 1952), and the one at Tecumseh, Mich., by the University of Michigan School of Public Health (Epstein *et al* 1965).

Some of these surveys have been limited in their objectives, but some are backed by extensive laboratory work on an entire population group—for example, a study of family experiences with upper respiratory illness. This investigation was carried on by Dingle and a team of his colleagues in a selected population of a university faculty in the city of Cleveland, Ohio (Dingle *et al.* 1964). It demonstrated factors that increased or decreased such rates of illness in this particular group. Another example, perhaps not as elaborate as the Cleveland study, is quoted on streptococcal pharyngitis and rheumatic fever in a Dutch village in chapter 15.

But the scope of most of these surveys lies a little outside the field of the average doctor, or even of an epidemiologically minded physician, whose dealings with the local population must of necessity be primarily confined to his own patients, representing as they do members of the local community who come to him for advice. In spite of the gradual disappearance of the family doctor from the medical scene, and regardless how unpopular the home visit may have become, the family remains a fundamental unit of importance for any physician who attempts to cultivate the clinical epidemiological approach. He can begin, for instance, by regarding the family of his patient as a domiciliary unit which can be considered in the same light as an individual case. It deserves a history, and an examination of as many members of the domicile as possible, an examination of the kindred, and an examination of the environment of the home.

THE FAMILY APPROACH

The family is the ideal unit to consider for epidemiological study because common hereditary and environmental conditions exist in a group of individuals, a domiciliary group living in intimate contact with one another whose members, for a certain time at least, are quite conscious of their common life. The term "family" is used here in a broad sense, and it includes the household, whether it be limited to a one-room apartment or to a farm with all its appurtenances, including animals and birds and their respective parasites—an epidemiologic situation in itself. The many examples of how disease tends to be aggregated or concentrated within household groups are familiar enough, but we hasten to state that, in spite of our emphasis so far on infectious disease, an aggregation of cases within the family group does not mean that the condition is infectious. Obviously certain hereditary defects may be concentrated within some families, such as hemophilia or syndactylism; or certain habits conditioned by the environment can affect all members of the family group, thus giving rise to an aggregation or clustering of cases caused by, for instance, a dietary deficiency such as pellagra.

So the physician can be in the front line here, and a beginning can be made without much expense or the necessity of a team of specialists. This is true whether the determining factor is genetic or environmental or both. Here the careful intimate study of the younger age groups in a particular kindred can be most rewarding. As for the environment, continued ecologic observations that include mapping of social climates should aid in revealing any abnormal exposures. It should also include records of the psychological reactions of individual members to adversity, illness, or trauma. Furthermore the physician is generally in the best position to bring timely therapeutic or preventive measures to bear.

But let us return, for purposes of emphasis, to a clustering of cases of a particular disease within the home. This may be due to multiple causes; to an infection, to a nutritional disturbance, or to habits that may be exceedingly important. The example of an infestation with body lice or scabies in a family is a case in point. The real basic defect in this family may be an innate tendency not to use soap and water. Thus the habits of the whole family are conditioned by heredity as well as by environment.

Using typhoid fever as another kind of example, the observations of Ramsey (1935) and Stebbins and Reed (1937) in New York state indicated that the probability of contracting typhoid was from 1,200 to 1,900 times greater in a familial associate of a patient with the disease than in the general population. Infectious hepatitis offers an example of a family outbreak in which a confusing element exists, for the infection may be so mild, particularly in the youngest members of the family, that only a careful clinical analysis with transaminase tests can reveal actual infection. Often the infantile cases of hepatitis are unrecognizable or unsuspected until a parent happens to acquire the overt, adult disease as a result of close association with the infectious, although apparently healthy, infant.

But a growing body of evidence testifies that of all the factors involved in familial clusters of disease, the genetic influence is probably the most pervasive. As Francis (1965) has said, "casual reflection leads to the realization that this survival cannot be attributed to any one item in our genetic code; rather the influences are multiple or polygenic. . . . So when the human geneticist turns to disease and disorder in the population as his basis of genetic analysis, he is promptly in epidemiology." (1965).

This takes us back to our original premise of the value of the family as a unit for clinical observation and care, and the desirability for taking advantage of this approach. Although the methods of examining a family are constantly changing and new and sophisticated techniques are being introduced each year, there is certainly little that is new about the family-doctor approach.

The role of the clinical epidemiologist is like that of a detective visiting the scene of the crime.[1] He starts with the examination of a sick individual and cautiously branches out into the setting where that individual became ill and where the patient may also become ill again. In this respect the clinical epidemiologist stands in relation to the statistical epidemiologist perhaps as a gardener does to a farmer. The statistician may validate his analyses by increasing the numbers of observations, whereas the clinician has the opportunity to complete the clinical picture and to improve the accuracy of a limited number of observations by intimate study and exacting measurements. This restriction of the size of the groups with which the clinical epidemiologist deals is certainly not essential, but is cultivated because clinical talents, exercised within the framework of an intimate doctor-patient relationship, cannot be readily applied wholesale without the risk of their being spread too thinly to be effective.

An example of this sort of detective work is found in the story of Zenker and trichinosis, which was a landmark in the epidemiology of that disease. Zenker noted the relationship between human trichinosis and trichinosis in the pig by the study of a single small outbreak, starting with a single patient. Part of the story, as related by Blumer (1939), can be found in a case report, recorded a century ago, of a twenty-year-old maid-servant

---

[1] This same chain of procedures has been found useful in teaching clinical epidemiology to third- and fourth-year medical students. The procedure recommended by some is to start the student at the bedside and lead him gradually away from it.

employed at an inn in Germany. She came to the hospital on January 12, 1860, having been ill since Christmas and having taken to her bed at the New Year with a fever that was thought for a while to be typhoid fever. She died on January 27, 1860.

At the autopsy, Zenker demonstrated great numbers of the parasites of trichinosis in the muscles. But his observations went farther than the autopsy table, for he took the trouble to go out to the inn where the patient had been employed. There he found that a hog had been slaughtered on the twenty-first of December. He was able to get samples of the meat from this hog, and in this tissue also, he found numerous encapsulated trichinae. He then learned that the wife of the landlord was sick at the same time as the maid, that her husband was sick later, and that the butcher who slaughtered the hog was also sick. He drew the conclusion that the infection of the sick persons was caused by the consumption of trichinous pork.

This is an example of clinical epidemiology in which an alert pathologist worked out the pathogenesis of an important disease by starting with one case. The discovery stemmed from an interest in details under which a patient became ill. By placing the patient in the setting whence her illness came, instead of regarding her as a lone sick individual who had suddenly popped out of a healthy setting, Zenker brought his pathological judgment to bear on the situation as well as on the patient. As a pathologist with his "workshop" in the hospital, he probably had as many reasons to remain immersed in his many duties there as modern pathologists have; yet he did not dispatch his laboratory assistant or a social worker to the home. Apparently he was ready and willing to venture out himself to the setting where the trouble actually arose.

This brief story is mentioned because modern medicine tends to concentrate on measurements and observations of sick people in an examining room, or in a hospital bed, where, for purposes of accuracy, patients are isolated from their usual surroundings, from their families, even stripped of their clothes. Unwittingly, the physician also isolates himself from the patients' surroundings by this procedure. This comment should not detract from the obvious fact that hospitalization has enormous advantages in the care of the sick. The hospital brings specialists together, it concentrates special facilities in one place, and it brings therapy to bear where and when it is needed most. Nevertheless, the point here is that hospital care is not the end of all modern clinical medicine, particularly if the science of preventive medicine is to be developed. And this development, in turn, depends a great deal upon the intelligent application of its basic science— epidemiology.

Again, it should be emphasized that the population involved need not be large for the study to be epidemiologic in scope. Actually an intimate study on a population of large size is almost impossible for one man to carry out, much less comprehend.

The most telling example I can give to illustrate the early work in clinical epidemiology on an infectious disease in which the laboratory was freely used was the program Dr. E. L. Opie undertook to study tuberculosis at the Henry Phipps Institute in Philadelphia in the 1920's. Dr. Opie temporarily forsook the career of an academic pathologist because he saw an opportunity to use certain new tools that had only recently become available to study tuberculosis. The tubercle bacillus had long before been discovered, but von Pirquet's tuberculin test, which that Viennese pediatrician brought to America in the early twentieth century, was relatively new and could stand more clinical testing. Opie's team of explorers carried out sequential tuberculin tests, sputum examinations and cultures, and chest x-rays. The chest x-ray was only beginning to be used routinely after World War I, and the family method of studying clusters or near-clusters of disease was just getting underway. It is commonplace today, in fact essential, to use these methods to study any domicile in which any member has tuberculosis, but it was not commonplace in the early 1920's. Perhaps Opie's most important contribution was the chart he devised for recording a chronological history of pertinent events, so that the spread of tuberculosis within families could be recorded in a new shorthand language.

The major value of the chart is that one can see at a glance the size of the family group, something about the health of all its members, the time relationships that certain events bear to illnesses, and time relationships between multiple familial illnesses. Furthermore, from these diagrams it can sometimes be demonstrated that, although an illness may have seemed to appear suddenly amid a healthy setting, the stage had been already set for days, weeks, or even months beforehand, and the sudden case happens to be the only one that has manifested itself and been recognized.

All this was accomplished in a few years. And Dr. Opie could go back to being an academic pathologist, leaving an enormous number of followers to develop his method in tuberculosis clinics (Puffer 1944).

The family chart has been used constantly to depict and clarify events not only of infectious but of noninfectious diseases including those of hereditary origin. One of the first such efforts was with rheumatic fever (Paul and Salinger 1931). This was a trial in the years before the microbial cause was known. At any event by this method it was clearly documented that within a "rheumatic family," [2] provided there were enough patients over six to eight years old, there was a clear demonstration that periods of rheumatic activity would sweep through the family in waves. Usually these waves would follow an epidemic of upper respiratory illness in the family, but not always.

Within a year, however, the bacterial (etiologic) agent of rheumatic fever was identified by the work of Coburn (1931), Schlesinger (1930), Bradley (1931), Glover and Griffith (1931). A great step forward had been achieved that was soon to be reflected in the therapeutic measures directed against rheumatic fever and later in prophylactic programs.

We have drawn upon another of our experiences with this approach to present the situation of a household outbreak of poliomyelitis, illustrated in Fig. 4. This occurred in the prevaccinal days of the 1930's, when poliomyelitis was regarded as a disease with a very low index of contagion and when textbook

---

[2] The definition of a rheumatic family was one in which two or more members had active or old evidences of rheumatic fever.

articles maintained that multiple infection in families was rare. In other words, the concept of inapparent infection, or abortive poliomyelitis, was infinitely less firmly established than it is now. This particular situation, with rapid intrafamilial spread of the disease is fundamental to our present ideas about poliomyelitis, now classified as having a high index of infection but a low index of paralytic cases. This is illustrated in the family chart drawn in 1937 (see Fig. 4). Here a case of paralytic poliomyelitis in the

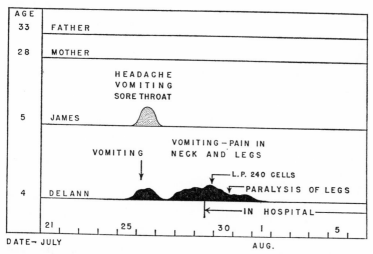

Fig. 4. A familial epidemic of poliomyelitis in prevaccinal days. The four individual members are represented by the horizontal lines; the respective ages of the children and their parents are given on the left. The period of time during which the family was under observation appears on the scale below. The black area roughly indicates the clinical course of a rather severe paralytic attack of poliomyelitis sustained by Del Ann. The stippled area represents the occurrence of a simultaneous minor illness thought at that time (July, 1931) to have nothing to do with Del Ann's illness until virus studies on the child James proved positive for poliovirus. (From Paul and Trask, 1932. *J. Exp. Med.* **56:**319.)

child Del Ann was recognized as an event of considerable clinical importance. A minor illness in her brother James was later proved to be abortive poliomyelitis. This second event was of little clinical importance to the physician or to the family, but it was of considerable consequence to the epidemiologist. In retrospect it is possible that other members of this family might have been involved in the familial epidemic, for the parents may have sustained inapparent infections with the family strain of poliovirus. The pattern of disease, shown in Fig. 4, has become much clearer since 1931. The usual spread of poliovirus infection within members of a family depends on a variety of conditions: the family environment, the ages of members, the individuals, their susceptibility to various serotypes of poliovirus, and the virulence of the strain. For instance, in a family having four or five juvenile susceptibles ranging from 3 to 12 years of age, one might consider the chances, estimated as percentages, of only one of the children acquiring paralysis at about 1 per cent; 3 to 6 per cent of the children might acquire abortive poliomyelitis or non-paralytic poliomyelitis, and more than 90 per cent, subclinical or inapparent infection with poliovirus. Who knows how many viral diseases have variants of this same pattern in greater or lesser degrees?

One could go on quoting examples of the clinical practice of epidemiology interminably, but I shall mention only a few more. One resulted from a visit in midwinter to the home of a very sick patient, who at that time was in the hospital suffering from an obscure type of pneumonia which eventually was fatal. Acting solely on the advice of a nine-year-old child, who was immediately punished by her parents for mentioning this fact, we poked around in the ash can at the back of the house and found a dead and frozen parrot. The diagnosis of psittacosis was not only made on this patient, but several other cases were unearthed, all of which had been acquired from the same bird. This episode occurred at a time when no cases of psittacosis had been recognized in the local area for at least fifteen years.

And, the discovery, after a long search, of a bottle of carbon tetrachloride in the bottom of a university hockey-player's locker can be cited. He had been suffering from a puzzling liver condition for two winters, had been seen by several specialists, and had already had a gall-bladder operation. It turned out that almost daily during the hockey season he had been washing his hands in this fluid (the nature or the name of which he did not know) to remove the stains of tire tape that had been applied to protect his knuckles.

As another example of the lines along which the epidemiologically minded physician might proceed, one can compare different points of view in the handling of a case of uncomplicated lobar (pneumococcus) pneumonia in a male adult thirty-five years old (see Fig. 5). To the curative physician this is an acute, serious illness, pneumonia with anemia. It demands immediate

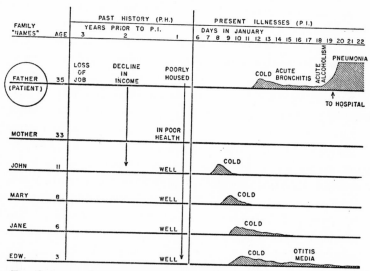

FIG. 5. A case of pneumonia in a 35-year-old adult and its relation to a few preceding events in the life of the patient and the life of his family. The six heavy horizontal lines indicate the six members who compose the family group. Their ages appear at the left of the diagram. The patient appears on the top line as the male parent of the family. The situation illustrated here culminated in a major illness in an individual who, either through bad luck or poor management, was in a somewhat vulnerable position for the contraction of pneumonia and might indeed be headed for future troubles.

medical treatment. The patient is removed to a hospital, and all efforts are directed toward a prompt cure with antibiotics and transfusions and, in keeping with modern hospital practices, a quick discharge of the patient to his home—an episode happily ended when the fever comes down and the hemoglobin restored to more normal levels. To the practitioner who is epidemiologically minded the case is still a pneumococcus infection in which all the above-mentioned procedures are indicated, but besides this the physician may wish to consider that this acute illness had been conditioned by a train of preceding events. Here his attitude may be no different from that of many a doctor who knows his families and the community well. In this particular case the history stated that the patient was married and had four children; he was a veteran and had been drawing some compensation for an old traumatic injury. He was not regularly employed, one of the reasons given, being that when he was employed the compensation he received from the government declined. To get ready money he had been acting as a professional blood donor almost weekly and this had brought his hemoglobin to about half its normal value. Recently he had exhibited a growing tendency to alcoholism, which had resulted in the neglect of his family, currently housed in poor and damp living quarters; indeed the whole family was at present suffering from an epidemic of colds or some type of acute upper respiratory infection. The patient, probably a victim of the family epidemic, also had contracted a cold and had attempted to cure it with alcohol. This resulted in a night on a park bench and pneumonia. According to this story, the pneumococcus is only the last invader in a chain of events.

The clinical epidemiologist or the practitioner of preventive medicine could not have altered a single detail of the events that led up to this particular case of pneumonia. But, having learned of these facts and written them into the case record, the doctor is in a better position to advise this patient at the time of his discharge from the hospital and subsequently.

In an attempt to get young physicians into the habit of acting on this principle of the family unit, the Yale University School of Medicine has used modifications of the domiciliary chart for teaching, clinical, and investigative purposes for more than 35 years, recording events in a variety of diseases: scarlet fever, enteroviral infections and upper respiratory viral diseases, and rheumatoid arthritis. Often a chart of the family has become an adjunct to the hospital history and has proved better than a long written history.

One could go on with a long series of other situations, some of which belong in the field of genetics, some in psychosomatic medicine, but all in medicine. All these situations call loudly for a doctor in the house, not necessarily as a dispenser of home care, but as a clinical investigator, in epidemiology if you will, intent upon factors which are related to the pathogenesis of disease or its prolongation. Such a doctor should be undisturbed by the fact that these situations call for a certain degree of pioneering that at least superficially, might seem to fall outside the province of ordinary medical practice.

Often the epidemiologist must set his own arbitrary standards to determine what manifestations of disease he is going to accept or measure, or what new measurements can be developed. For instance, if an hereditary condition is suspected, one can begin by searching in the kindred for overt cases as well as in those members who exhibit traces that only can be detected by appropriate laboratory determinations. Or, if the disease is an infectious one such as tuberculosis, how different the prevalence figures in a given family or any population would be if one recorded the various rates at which the group showed: (*a*) sputum positive for tubercle bacilli, (*b*) positive chest x-rays, and (*c*) positive tuberculin tests. Actually it would be informative to have all three of these rates recorded for a given series of families covering a period of several years. One would then have, for prevalence considerations, the open, serious cases, the mild cases, and the subclinical cases. The case rate would be one thing and the infection rate another. This principle applies to many diseases.

A fundamental difference between the methods of the epidemiologist and those of the clinician is that the former is apt to use rates rather than a series of cases. The epidemiologist must devise his own means of determining how common various representative pictures of a given disease may be. Often he may include the numbers of inapparent or subclinical cases of a given disease that are of no importance to the therapeutist but of

45

extreme importance to the epidemiologist. He must also take time to define the limits of the population at risk, and its size. This will give him the denominator:

$$\frac{\text{Number of cases (clinical or inapparent)}}{\text{population at risk}} = \text{rate.}$$

Having finally assembled data for this ratio, he can begin to consider seriously the circumstances within a given family group or community under which the varying rates of overt or inapparent illness have occurred.

THE COMMUNITY CHART

It would be a painstaking task to attempt to make a series of family charts of a community involving more than fifty or sixty people, and to compute rates therefrom. The labor involved might well be too great to make the study worthwhile. Nevertheless, in certain compact communities or institutions, a diagrammatic scheme of this same general type has proved to be of considerable value, along with spot maps, chronological charts, and so forth, but these techniques go beyond the scope of this chapter.

BIBLIOGRAPHY

BLUMER, G. 1939. Some remarks on the early history of trichinosis (1822–1866). *Yale J. Biol. Med.* 11:581.

BORDLEY, J. 1950. The hospital in the rural community. *Trans. Coll. Physicians, Phila. 4 Ser.* 18:56–64.

COBURN, A. 1931. *The factor of infection in the rheumatic state.* Baltimore: Williams & Wilkins Co.

DAWBER, T. R. and KANNEL, W. B. Susceptibility to coronary heart disease. 1961. Modern concepts of cardiovascular disease, 30:671–76.

DINGLE, J. H., BADGER, G. F., and JORDAN, W. S. 1964. *Illness in the home. A study of 25,000 illnesses in a group of Cleveland families.* Cleveland: Western Reserve University Press.

DOWNES, J. 1950. Cause of illness among males and females. *Milbank Mem. Fund Quart.* 27:No. 4.

———. 1952. The longitudinal study of families as a method of research. In *Research in public health.* New York: Milbank Memorial Fund.

EPSTEIN, F. H., FRANCIS, T., HAYNER, N. S., JOHNSON, B. J., KJELS-
BERG, M. O., NAPIER, J. A., OSTRANDER, L. D., PAYNE, M. W., and
DODGE, H. J. 1965. Prevalence of chronic diseases and distribution
of selected physiologic variables in a total community, Tecumseh,
Michigan. *Am. J. Epidemiology* 81:307–22.

FRANCIS, T. 1965. Genetics and epidemiology. Opening comments in
genetics and the epidemiology of chronic diseases, pp. 1–6. U.S.
Dept. Health, Education, and Welfare. Washington, D.C.: Government Printing Office.

GENETICS and the epidemiology of chronic diseases. 1965. Pp. 1–395.
U.S. Dept. Health, Education, and Welfare. Washington, D.C.:
Government Printing Office.

GLOVER, J. A., and GRIFFITH, F. 1931. Acute tonsillitis and some of
its sequels: Epidemiological and bacteriological observations. *Brit.
Med. J.* 2:521.

MACKENZIE, J. 1922–26. *Reports of the St. Andrews Institute for
Clinical Research.* Vols. I–III. London: Oxford University Press.

OPIE, E. L., and MCPHEDRAN, F. M. 1926. Spread of tuberculosis
within families. *J.A.M.A.* 87:1549.

PAUL, J. R. and SALINGER, R. 1931. The spread of rheumatic fever
through families. *J. Clin. Invest.* 9:33–51.

———— and TRASK, J. D. 1932. The detection of poliomyelitis virus
in so-called abortive types of the disease. *J. Exp. Med.* 56:319–43.

PICKLES, W. N. 1939. *Epidemiology in country practice.* Baltimore:
Williams & Wilkins Co.

PUFFER, RUTH, R. 1944. *Familial susceptibility to tuberculosis.* Cambridge: Harvard University Press.

RAMSEY, G. H. 1935. Typhoid fever among household contacts with
special reference to vaccination. *Am. J. Hyg.* 21:665.

SMUTS, J. C. 1926. *Holism and evolution.* New York: Macmillan Co.

SPENCE, J. C., WALTON, W. S., MILLER, F. J. W. and COURT, S. D. M.
1954. *A thousand families in New Castle-upon-Tyne.* London, Oxford University Press.

————. 1950. Family studies in preventive pediatrics. *New Engl.
J. Med.* 243:205.

STEBBINS, E. L. and REED, E. 1937. Carrier-borne typhoid fever in
New York State with special reference to attack rates among household contacts. *Am. J. Pub. Health* 27:233.

TRUSSELL, R. E. 1955. *Hunterdon medical center.* Cambridge: Harvard University Press.

CHAPTER V

Concepts of Etiology: The Seed, the Soil, and the Climate

Behold, a sower went forth to sow;
And when he sowed, some seeds fell by the way side, and the fowls came and devoured them up.
Some fell upon stony places, where they had not much earth: and forthwith they sprung up, because they had no deepness of earth:
And when the sun was up, they were scorched; and because they had no root, they withered away.
And some fell among thorns; and the thorns sprung up, and choked them:
But others fell into good ground, and brought forth fruit, some one hundred-fold, some sixty-fold, some thirty-fold.

Matt. 13:3–8

The above quotation from Scripture reminds us that the farmer requires good *seed*, good *soil*, and a proper *climate*, if his crops are to be plentiful. These agricultural similes can be applied by the epidemiologist to processes that give rise to disease, although it may seem strange to compare a bountiful crop with a sizable epidemic.

Busy practicing physicians tend to seek simple explanations when it comes to a decision about what causes a disease. They tend to regard at least two of our three categories—the soil and the climate—as influences rather than causes. Academic epidemiologists, conversely, would be more likely to regard all three as causes. Somewhere between the two stands the clinical epidemiologist. In any event such "secondary causes" as genetic factors or ways of living seldom appear in a patient's routine hospital record unless the physician gives special thought to it.

But it is likely that more and more attention will be paid to such causes in the future. And by extending the boundaries of the physician's thought and action beyond the consulting room, ward, and clinic, epidemiology "provides a third dimension to the understanding of disease by creating awareness of the nature of the environment in which disability arises, of the factors in the community which contribute to its causation and, in turn its effect upon the community" (Francis 1954). Returning then to the agricultural simile of the seed, the soil, and the climate, we find that, in the course of medical education and practice, a vast amount of emphasis has been placed on the first of these, understandably enough, and much less on the other two.

The Seed

An etiological agent represents to most of us something that is tangible, whether it be a virus, a bacterium, a plasmodium, or a chemical or physical agent. In the case of a virulent pathogenic micro-organism it receives first priority. Both microbiology and parasitology as applied to human and animal diseases are deeply concerned with it. But the agent may be a chemical poisoning, or physical trauma, or carcinogens of both known and unknown nature. Other potential agents of damage that precipitate accidents and injury include the roller skate carelessly left at the head of the stairs or the automobile traveling at the rate of seventy miles an hour. It is enough to say that innumerable direct causative agents of disease or injury are known to exist, and no doubt there are many unknown to us today. They all operate within a given situation or framework. Their study embraces a variety of different fields.

For the sake of simplicity, it may be easier to discuss this complex situation by limiting our considerations for the moment to infectious diseases where it is generally customary to reduce the etiology of a given infection to a single infectious agent, although, as already emphasized, this often turns out to be an oversimplification. Before Pasteur, it was felt that infectious disease was often caused by a concatenation of circumstances, in the midst of which the idea of *contagium vivum* occupied a small although conceivably vital role—an idea that does not seem to be so far from correct today. In the late nineteenth century, however, as the science of bacteriology developed, the concept of multiple etiologic factors rapidly gave way to that of a single cause. The medical profession has more or less retained this attitude ever since.

In this present age of antibiotics, multiple causes of an infectious disease do not appeal as much to clinicians, who are constantly trying to find that weak link in the chain of events that leads to infection, that is, the link that can be most readily broken. Attacking the bacterial agent with antibiotics is the most effective way. Not only does such an attack on the microbe sometimes cure the patient, it may even curtail the spread of the microbe within the community, as has been demonstrated with streptococcal infections and certain venereal diseases. So it is understandable that physicians still concentrate their efforts on the parasite as the key to the whole situation. To students also, starting out on their medical studies, it is an acceptable and even comforting idea that the cause of a disease, presumably a noxious agent, can be captured and kept in a test tube, isolated so that it can be tested for its virulence and its sensitivity to antibiotics, as well as for its capacity to be made into antigens useful for diagnosis and immunization. Indeed, it is a general truth that only those factors that can be separated and accurately measured have a satisfying meaning for the student of science, whether he be young or old.

Nevertheless, after the idea of the single cause had been ridden hard for two generations, it came to be regarded, by epidemiologists at least, as an oversimplification. It takes more than a microbe to produce a disease, just as it takes more than a seed to produce a plant. Microbiology and epidemiology are not the same discipline nor have they been considered so since Pettenkofer's day. It falls to the epidemiologist to discover things, other than a single etiologic agent, that he might hope to measure and put in their proper places as factors contributing to the initiation and maintenance of a given disease. It becomes his responsibility, so to speak, to differentiate direct precipitating causes from supplementary causes and to assign them priorities. These other causes are to be found in the characteristics of individual members of the population attacked, as well as in the environments in which both host and parasite find themselves. It is the sum or interaction of these influences that gives rise to disease.

The reason for laboring this point here is that it is often difficult, and even arbitrary, to decide whether a person infected is ill or not, and accessory factors may swing the balance in a favorable or unfavorable direction. Thus, almost no one has ever regarded the tubercle bacillus as being the one and only cause of tuberculosis. Tubercle bacilli are important in a situation where host resistance and environmental conditions also play etiologic roles. The latter determine not only whether the host (or potential patient) acquires the infection but also whether the infection will be severe enough to cause illness. The carrier of pneumococci is, in a sense, an infected person. If he has a cold and subsequently falls through the ice during the winter, and his mild infection gets worse and develops into pneumococcal pneumonia, the pneumococcus is actually no more solely responsible for his illness than is winter weather. Indeed, the exposure of a susceptible or a non-immune person to a bacterium or a virus may, under certain circumstances, be a completely negative event; or it may result in an inapparent (subclinical) infection that can actually be a salutary experience for the host, giving him an added degree of immunity without the price of illness. An infection may result, however, that even can prove fatal.

It becomes very apparent, therefore, that there are contributory factors determining whether a given etiologic agent will produce a severe disease, a mild disease, or none at all. And it becomes a matter of opinion whether these contributory factors are designated as multiple causes or supplementary factors. Certainly they deserve recognition by physicians although their importance varies in degree, and even more certainly, they deserve not only the attention of the epidemiologist but careful measurement by him.

THE SOIL

Man's resistance, conditioned from both hereditary and environmental standpoints, occupies a dominant position in determining whether he will acquire a certain disease. This brings us to a consideration of the next item of our agricultural simile, the soil. The soil here is the human or animal host and its condition at the time the seed is sown (provided the seed is actually necessary, for indeed in certain hereditary developmental conditions it would appear it is not). To the clinician so-called host factors represent man's susceptibility—his ability to cope with or to succumb to infection, injury, or any kind of insult.

Genetic influences are major host factors (*Genetics and the Epidemiology of Chronic Diseases* 1965). Actually they pervade every corner of man's susceptibility, and there is an increasing awareness of their significance, as is evident from the development of divisions of medical genetics in the curriculum of medical schools within the past few years. The relationship of inherited tendencies to susceptibility to specific disease just as for other disease-producing tendencies, can generally be presented on a spectrum. McKusick (1965) has presented such a spectrum, arbitrarily assigning the places of greatest genetic susceptibility to phenylketonuria and galactosemia, and those least susceptible to hypertension, peptic ulcer, and tuberculosis.

There are innumerable aspects of this hereditary pattern of susceptibility such as predispositions of certain races or even families to disease, and the blood-group and disease associations. Mammalian susceptibility to a bacterial or viral disease in mice is discussed in the next chapter on experimental epidemiology and selective breeding or eugenics—if that is the word for it in animals. Another aspect of man's vulnerability represents the sum total of what has been called in military parlance his "seasoning experiences." Most of these experiences represent natural exposure to viruses, bacteria, or other parasites, although closely related are courses of artificial immunizations which all go to make up the phenotype. At least the host can react to influences or injury, whether acquired knowingly or unknowingly, that do not invoke immune mechanisms as we know them. Certainly infection does not have to produce antibodies to render that host immune, but the process probably leaves some mark, temporary or permanent, on him that we can sometimes measure. Although, inevitably, in dealing with the intricacies of host resistance we have had to emphasize factors that we cannot comprehend, we are in a much better position than we were a generation ago. Some kinds of host resistance are becoming more subject to measurement. The use of skin tests (Schick and tuberculin test surveys) on a mass basis, and the new uses of serological epidemiology (see chap. 13), which are being explored, do represent useful measures of man's resistance to infectious disease that can be employed on a large scale. Scores of new

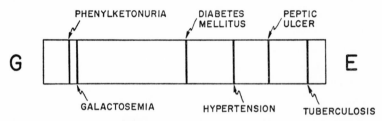

Fig. 6. Schematic representation of spectrum on which several diseases are listed with regard to the relative importance of genetic and environmental factors in pathogenesis. (After McKusick, V. A., 1965. Coronary artery disease. In: *Genetics and the epidemiology of chronic diseases.* U.S. Public Health Service. Publication No. 1163, p. 134. Washington, D.C.: Government Printing Office.)

antibody tests have been devised in the past two decades, but other blood components such as blood lipids, blood enzymes, and factors of nutritional importance can be measured in today's serum surveys.

Furthermore there are a great variety of ways in which one can treat the soil—nutritional therapy, replacement measures, hormone therapy, and so forth. The increasing use of ACTH and cortisone in the treatment of a variety of diseases, as well as that of other hormones and vitamins, are additional examples. And when it comes to prophylactic measures to be employed before the seed is sown, various immunization procedures represent examples of "pretreatment of the soil" to render it unreceptive to the seed.

THE CLIMATE

A third factor is the environment to which seed and soil are exposed. Obviously, there is much that cannot be measured here. It has been said that epidemiology has no more right to be considered an exact science than has meteorology. Both deal with nebulous things. But at least epidemiological climates can be divided into two parts, macroclimate and microclimate. Macroclimate is climate in the ordinary meteorological sense—temperature, rainfall, humidity, and so on. Microclimate is the sum of those intimate living conditions and ways of life representing the socioeconomic or domiciliary conditions in which a given individual finds himself, which effect his exposure to illness and condition his resistance against it. It includes rural or urban living, housing, temperature and humidity within the home or working place, living space, sanitation, food, and all the circumstances of poverty or affluence. Poor housing and crowding can thus become just as important, even dominant, in the causation of upper respiratory infections as viruses or pneumococci. The aftermath of war and all its attendant circumstances produces microclimates in which famine, tuberculosis, and epidemic typhus may rise and flourish. Such features will be dealt with later in this book, but it should be emphasized here that the climate does not act solely on the host,—obviously it acts on the parasite or its vectors as well.

When these various factors, paraphrased in terms of the simile of seed, soil, and climate, are considered together, it becomes a little clearer how each of them can exert some related influence upon the pathogenesis of a given disease.

BIBLIOGRAPHY

FRANCIS, T. 1954. The teaching of epidemiology, *J. Med. Educ.* **29:** 15.

Genetics and the Epidemiology of chronic diseases. 1965. U.S. Department of Health, Education, and Welfare. Public Health

Service Publication No. 1163. Washington, D.C.: Government Printing Office.

McKusick, V. A. 1965. Coronary artery disease in genetics and the epidemiology of chronic diseases. In *Genetics and the epidemiology of chronic diseases*. U.S. Department of Health Education, and Welfare. Public Health Service Publication No. 1163. Washington, D.C.: Government Printing Office, pp. 133–43.

PART II

Methods and Uses

Experimental Epidemiology

Although considerable emphasis has been placed in this book upon the idea that the principles of modern epidemiology can be applied to all types of illness, or even injuries, it is infectious disease that is continually stressed, because this kind of illness represents a natural introduction to the general concepts of epidemiology. It is also in the field of infectious disease that experimental methods on a large scale can and have been used to advantage—a discipline which has been called experimental epidemiology.[1] Such experiments employing mice began a generation ago when W. W. C. Topley in England pointed out that one way to solve some of the major problems in epidemiology was "to turn our backs on the natural world, and to simplify our conditions until the number of variable factors reached manageable proportions, and then to see what happens when we hold some factors constant and vary others" (Topley, 1942, p. 337).

Topley achieved this objective fairly satisfactorily; over a period of twenty-five years he conducted a series of observations in the field of experimental epidemiology that will probably remain classics for some time. During this same period in the United States, L. T. Webster (1946) of the Rockefeller Institute for Medical Research was also active in developing this new science. Students of epidemiology owe some debt to these men in particular. It is unfortunate that both died before their programs

---

[1] It should not be surmised however, that modern experimental epidemiology need be limited in scope to the study of infections. The action of poisons on populations of mice or rats, or physical agents or inadequate diets that threaten the health or lives of living things, can all be included in this discipline, but infectious disease willl be stressed in this chapter.

were completed, for much remains to be done, not only with infectious but with non-infectious diseases.

Primary questions with which these investigators were concerned were: What are the factors which initiate epidemics? What prolongs them and what brings them to an end? How do they maintain themselves in a community, in the face of man's prodigious efforts to stamp out the infection? In such studies it is presumed that something is known about how a given infection spreads from one individual to another before the experimental epidemiologist begins his work. From the study of a small group of not more than three or four animals, the experimentalist can subsequently branch out to consider how a larger group of exposed individuals becomes infected or escapes infection. This larger group, in epidemiological parlance, is often spoken of as the "herd" or, more aptly, the "herd at risk." We deal here as elsewhere with the relative importance of the three factors—seed, soil, and climate.

The presence of immunity in the herd is of obvious importance in conditioning the epidemiological behavior of various infections within various populations. Type 1 epidemics occur in susceptible populations, so-called virgin populations, exposed for the first time to a virulent infectious agent. Type 2 epidemics occur in populations within which the virulent organism is already established.

What is unknown, more difficult to predict or measure, is why some of the exposed individuals become ill, even fatally, and others, presumably equally exposed, are mildly infected or escape altogether. We also wonder why the epidemic comes to an end without involving the entire susceptible population. Is it a matter of the number of susceptible individuals or the dosage of the infectious agent? Did the virulence of the agent change during the epidemic? Did certain fortunate individuals become immunized as a result of subclinical infection during the early stages of the epidemic? Or are other factors, not yet recognized, involved?

Examples of Type 2 epidemics are the seasonal outbreaks of measles, whooping cough, or poliomyelitis that generally involve juveniles in urban surroundings. They are apt to be endemic within a semi-immune population that periodically becomes subject to outbreaks, presumably because a new and large enough crop of susceptibles is born and grows up between epidemics. But we do not know where the infective agents remain during interepidemic periods; and whether the properties of these causative infective agents are stable or mutate at certain times, allowing a relatively quiescent parasite to multiply extensively and spread throughout a population, inciting a vastly greater number of cases of the particular disease than the normal incidence. Probably each infection or disease is a law unto itself.

One hypothesis explaining the genesis of epidemics is that mutation in the causative microbial agent takes place during the period between epidemics or perhaps in the immediate pre-epidemic period, and this series of conditioned changes results in increased virulence that progresses until the epidemic has burned itself out. Another hypothesis is that the epidemic arises either because immunity had begun to decline in the exposed population or herd, or because the number of susceptibles had increased, giving rise to a situation that invites infection. A third explanation is, of course, that a change in the environment, such as a breakdown of sanitary facilities, might easily lead to a sudden increased dosage of the inciting organism. Indeed, a variety of host and environmental factors, including poor diet or at least a change in diet, or poor housing facilities might affect the population adversely by lowering its resistance as well as increasing its exposure.

These circumstances can be partially tested by experimental arrangements. Attempts were made by Topley and Webster to attack first the relationship of the fluctuating virulence of inciting microbes—the "mutation hypothesis"—to the genesis and decline of epidemics. Their observations and conclusions, particularly those of Webster, were limited largely to diseases caused by bacteria, as opposed to those caused by viruses.

That properties of bacteria, notably virulence, fluctuate has long been familiar to bacteriologists, who found they could reduce virulence by prolonged cultivation of bacteria on certain laboratory media and could often restore it by repeated passage through susceptible animals. It was suspected that in nature, too, virulence must fluctuate; if so, then this fluctuation provided a reasonable explanation for the rise and fall of epidemics. Nevertheless, Topley and Webster started with the premise that this mutation hypothesis was unproved, at least for the agents they employed.

The native diseases of mice that they studied included mouse typhoid, due to *Salmonella typhimurium, Salmonella enteritidis;* and a native respiratory infection due to *Bacillus Friedländeri;* and, by Topley, a virus infection due to ectromelia virus. In most of the early experiments an epidemic was started among a group of mice of predetermined age and size confined within a fixed amount of space, and the rate of progression of the epidemic was carefully observed. Later, space and various other factors, such as temperature and diets, were altered. The basic pattern could often be expressed in a simple graph, such as the one in Fig. 7.

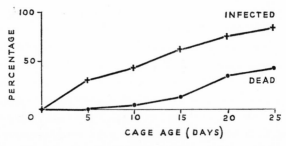

Fig. 7. Two graphs representing the rates at which 90 mice from a single herd became infected when exposed experimentally to mouse typhoid under controlled conditions. (From Topley, W. W. C., 1942. *Proc. Roy. Soc. Ser. B.* **130:**337.)

The experiment here indicates that under uniform conditions, using a special strain of the infecting organism, one could expect that at the end of a given period, a certain number of infected mice would have died, a certain number would have become sick and yet would recover, and a few others would not have shown any evidence of illness. In spite of the uniform age and stock of mice, however, the response of individual animals was not uniform; some mice died promptly after the minimum incubation period of six days, others died at varying periods up to twenty-five days and sometimes longer. An important point, however, was that this group response was found to be regular and predictable when batches of twenty or more mice were employed and when the infecting strain of bacterial microorganisms was kept the same; a difference in mortality rates could be expected from different strains of enteritides bacilli. Furthermore, it was equally important to hold constant the ages of the mice to be infected. Mice of unknown ages obtained from various different sources, with different experiences, and frequently infested with parasites or other infectious agents did not give this predictable pattern of results. In spite of these variables, the evidence was that certain factors were sufficiently stable so that a reproducible pattern of results could be obtained.

Granted, therefore, that a reproducible pattern could be obtained, Webster was able to compare simultaneously the virulence of *S. typhimurium* cultures derived from a strain of the bacteria cultured from the blood of acute cases of mouse typhoid just before death with that of cultures from the stools of healthy survivors. He found no differences. The same results were obtained when bacteremic and nasal carrier strains of Friedländer pneumonia organisms were compared. Titrations were also conducted on cultures of organisms recovered from populations of mice during various epidemic and endemic phases of infection. These tests revealed no differences in the epidemic or disease-producing capacity of these bacteria obtained from animals either during the height of the epidemic or during interepidemic periods. One might conclude, therefore, that *in these infections* and within the framework of the experiment, fluctuations in the virulence of these particular infecting bacteria, which had previously been thought responsible for the rise and decline of epidemics, could not be demonstrated.

Webster concluded that his results indicated a constant and fixed disease-producing power in certain given strains of organisms under the controlled conditions of host and environment that he tested. He believed levels of virulence might remain stable for years and was impressed with the dominant role of the host in determining epidemics. Topley was inclined to agree in part with this contention but was unwilling to admit that fluctuations in virulence never occurred, and that these fluctuations were not a natural cause of the genesis or decline of epidemics. What they had proved was that the virulence of the microbic organisms might remain fixed, and yet epidemics could be produced and could decline by varying other factors that concerned both the herd and its environment.

It should again be emphasized that these were specialized experiments illustrating a given principle that is occasionally operative, and the results cannot be immediately projected into a series of generalizations or epidemiological laws. Most of this work was done twenty years ago, and nearly all of it dealt with a small number of bacterial diseases; in fact, only one viral infection was included. Today much new information is available. Indeed, we know that certain bacteria or viruses, not tested in Webster's experiments, can actually undergo a change *in vivo*, which may or may not have anything to do with the epidemic potentialities of these strains. Rammelkamp and his co-workers (1952) observed that in men acutely infected with a given type of Group A hemolytic streptococci, this organism frequently lost one of its components (the so-called M substance) while harbored in the throats of patients during convalescence.

It is strongly suspected also that *in vivo* transformations among certain subtypes of influenza viruses A, A ^{1}, and B can occur in nature. As a result of this phenomenon, a new subtype can arise and can actually be responsible for outbreaks; but whether this "mutant" virus undergoes fluctuations during the decline of epidemics or when it is forced to multiply within an immune human population is a matter that awaits further investigation. The disappointment in the efficiency of a reliable influenza vaccine which can be used year after year, has been ascribed to variability of the strain of influenza virus responsible for each particular epidemic.

Once a certain degree of stability of the infecting agent has been established, however, one should logically seek to measure, on the basis of this background, other factors which might enormously influence the situation. One can well imagine that under conditions of extreme crowding and extremes of temperature, the mortality of the exposed population of mice will increase. The effect of diet on an infection is most complex, depending upon the type of infecting organism being tested and the degree of malnutrition of the host. With some infections, surprisingly enough, if the host animal is deficient, the superimposed infection is less severe. This has been demonstrated, particularly with viral diseases: foot-and-mouth disease and vaccinia infections, pneumonia virus of mice (P. V. M.), and mouse-adapted poliovirus (Lansing strain).

The effect of poor diet often works in a detrimental way, however. Webster and his colleagues demonstrated that under certain circumstances those mice that had received a less adequate diet than others did not withstand natural or native enteric (bacterial) infection as well as did those that had received a better diet. This effect was not easily demonstrable and seemed to depend on the genetic constitution of the strain of mice employed. In clinical experience, nevertheless, the universal unfavorable effect of malnutrition on the clinical course of tuberculosis is recognized.

Turning from the climate to the soil, or herd resistance, it appears that immunity can obviously be of more than one kind: a natural, innate, or inherited capacity to succumb to or resist infection; a similar capacity, induced or maintained by a variety of local environmental conditions (including natural or artificial immunization), or other poorly understood factors. All may play some part in inhibiting the spread of a given infection through a given population. Probably the major contribution of experimental epidemiologists was to point out that inherited resistance played such an important part in any group of animals in which an experimental infection or epidemic had been induced.

The inherent capacity to resist infection was perhaps first put to practical use half a century ago. Early in the twentieth century, the resistance of particular strains of wheat to certain plant diseases was shown to be dependent upon a single-factor type of inheritance with susceptibility or resistance dominant. These observations were later extended to other plants. Workers studying infectious disease in animals apparently paid little attention to this until some years later. Here, although the situation was admittedly quite complex, experiments indicated that the resistance of animals to bacterial infections differed from their resistance to viral infections. That one could breed strains of mice both susceptible and resistant to bacterial infection is apparent from the data in Fig. 8, taken from

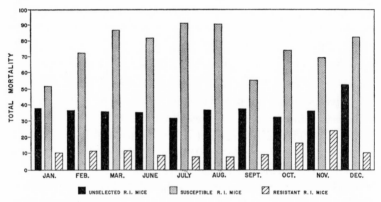

Fɪɢ. 8. Comparative mortalities carried out over a 12-month period on unselected and selected R. I. (Rockefeller Institute) mice following intrastomachal instillation of *Sal. enteritidis* (mouse typhoid) bacilli. (From Webster, L. T., 1946. Experimental epidemiology. *Medicine* **25:**77.)

Webster's monograph. Webster measured the comparative mortalities of unselected and selected mice after the intrastomachal instillation of *S. enteritidis*. The essential conclusion was that variability in host resistance and its regulation by inborn factors have considerable bearing on the spread and acquisition of infectious diseases, and, like acquired immunity, the variability could be measured. It was further noted that hereditarily resistant mice did not possess levels of specific antibodies higher than normal.

One of the most valuable contributions made by experimental

epidemiologists has been observing the spread and degree of a Type 2 epidemic by conducting experiments on a mixed population of mice, composed of hereditary susceptible and resistant animals. The experiments were done according to various techniques. In one of them, a constant number of susceptible and/or resistant mice was added to the infected colony each day for many months and even for several years. The addition of susceptible mice to infected herds containing chronic intestinal carriers of enteritides bacilli and residual members resistant to this infection tended to prolong the "epidemic period"; the addition of genetically resistant mice had the opposite effect. When the number of susceptible mice added each day, or week, was small, the death rate in the infected population showed wide and regular fluctuations with occasional intermissions. But not until there was a certain percentage of susceptibles in the herd at risk did the number of fatal cases rise to epidemic proportions. At no time in this particular series of experiments was it possible to demonstrate fluctuations in the virulence of the organisms responsible for the sporadic or epidemic infections.

In spite of my repeated warnings, I cannot resist the temptation to point out how the situation in human populations, notably in training camps for recruits, may resemble the experiments in some of these mouse populations. A characteristic situation can easily be imagined in a large camp of more or less fixed size, consisting of men who remain in the camp for variable periods of time, and into which groups of new recruits are admitted at a rate of several hundred each week to replace a similar number of departing "graduates." If the environment is appropriate for the spread of upper respiratory diseases in the camp, then a so-called Type 2 epidemic situation exists here, and as in the mouse experiments, it involves the introduction of susceptible "immigrants" into an area of endemic infections. An epidemic of upper respiratory infection lasting for quite a long time could result, and theoretically, if the increments kept coming and the environmental conditions remained the same, it could last indefinitely!

Furthermore it has become apparent in recent years that large scale observations on experimental epidemiology can be made with impunity on human subjects by using a harmless strain to infect them, i.e., one that has been attenuated. As an outstanding example, one can cite observations that have been possible since the vaccine strains of attenuated polioviruses were introduced and used in clinical trials. These strains, which began to be used in the late 1950's, have been employed increasingly since that date. There seems to be little difference (other than that of neurovirulence) between vaccine strains of attenuated polioviruses and of wild strains, except that the attenuated have a slightly reduced tendency to spread when introduced into a community (Fox *et al* 1961, p. 368). Yet apart from the standpoint of the strain's reduced capacity to infect by the usual route, both groups of strains are comparable. Both produce antibodies to the same degree. This enables one to make experimental observations on various features of the inapparent infection, such as the incubation period, the period of viremia (Horstmann *et al.* 1963), periods of nasopharyngeal and alimentary carriage of the virus (Horstmann *et al.* 1959), and on infection rates and conditions that favor the natural dissemination of the virus within and outside of family domiciles. Such observations can also include the rate and degree of development of antibodies in the test population, even the associated vector rate in the local fly and cockroach population, and the degree of contamination of local urban sewage with attenuated poliovirus strains (Riordan *et al.* 1961). These features can be observed and measured in relation to the local conditions when only a few individuals (vaccinees) are included in the test population, or when mass community vaccination campaigns are conducted.

An immense amount of new data and new knowledge has been accumulated by this new and informative method of experimental observation, which is a pure example of clinical experimental epidemiology. To a lesser extent, live measles-virus vaccine strains can serve as test models for what happens in the natural disease. The future is bright for this kind of clinical investigation in the field of epidemiology. By and large, though much more difficult, it is much more informative to see what happens in men than mice.

BIBLIOGRAPHY

Fox, J. P., Gelfand, H. M., LeBlanc, D. R., Potash, L., Clemmer, D. I. and LaPenta, D. 1961. The spread of vaccine strains of poliovirus in the household and in the community in southern Louisiana. In *Poliomyelitis. Papers and discussions presented at 5th International Poliomyelitis Conference.* Philadelphia: J. B. Lippincott Co.

Greenwood, M., Hill, B., A., Topley, W. W. C., and Wilson, J. 1936. Experimental epidemiology. *Spec. Rep. Ser. No. 209.* London: Medical Research Council.

Horstmann, D. M., Niederman, J. C. and Paul, J. R. 1959. Attenuated Type I poliovirus vaccine. Its capacity to infect and to spread from "vaccinees" within an institutional population. *J.A.M.A.* **170**:1–3.

Horstmann, D. M., Opton, E. M., Klemperer, R., Llado, B. and Vignec, A. J. 1964. Viremia in infants vaccinated with oral poliovirus vaccine (Sabin). *Am. J. Hyg.* **79**:47–63.

Horstmann, D. M., Niederman, J. C., Riordan, J. T., and Paul, J. R. 1959. The trial use of Sabin's attenuated Type I poliovirus vaccine in a village in Southern Arizona. *Amer. J. Hyg.* **70**:169–84.

Rammelkamp, C. H., Houser, H. B., Hahn, E. O., Wannamaker, L. W., Denny, F. W., and Echardt, G. C. 1952. The prevention of rheumatic fever. In *Rheumatic fever: a symposium,* ed. L. Thomas. Minneapolis: University of Minnesota Press.

Riordan, J. T., Paul, J. R., Yoshioka, I., and Horstmann, D. M. 1961. The detection of poliovirus and other enteric viruses in flies. Results of tests carried out during an oral poliovirus vaccine trial. *Am. J. Hyg.* **74**:123–36.

Topley, W. W. C. 1942. The biology of epidemics. *Proc. Roy. Soc., B* **130**:337.

Webster, L. T. 1946. Experimental epidemiology. *Medicine* **25**:77.

CHAPTER VII

Methods and Terms
I. Mortality Rates

We have stressed frequently that the approach to our subject
is to be from the standpoint of a clinician. Clinicians are used to
dealing with individual patients or their families. Epidemiologists, on the other hand, have nearly always dealt with rates of
illness in a group as opposed to individual patients. Sometimes it
is difficult for clinicians in general to spread their attentions thin
enough to cover large groups of people or, at least, to make this
transition readily from the individual to the community. The
practice of clinical epidemiology does not necessarily imply that
it will deal with relatively small groups and not with the large
populations which health officers, on either a local or national
scale, must handle. Regardless of the size of the group, however,
the epidemiologist, if he is to gain a proper idea of the frequency
of disease, always has to deal with a ratio:

$$\frac{\text{cases}}{\text{population}}$$

Within a group or community of any size, the general vital
statistics can have little significance unless they are related to the
actual number of people comprising the community under
surveillance. If the rates are to be meaningful, the measurements
of both numerator and denominator on which they rest must be
reasonably accurate. Only under such circumstances can they
have significance to the scientist.[1]

[1] In the following chapters and indeed elsewhere in this book the reader
is urged to use supplementary biostatistical texts. I recommend Bradford
Hill's *Statistical Methods in Clinical and Preventive Medicine* (1962).

Before going on to discuss the various techniques of measuring disease frequency, it may be well to define the terminology used in expressing the frequency with which a given disease or cause of death occurs in a given group. Common usage has often confused the meaning of *incidence* in contrast to *prevalence;* and since these familiar terms express separate aspects of morbidity, the sooner the attempt is made to differentiate between them, the better. Frequency measurements in an acute disease from which individuals may recover completely and that may give a lasting immunity are apt to be different from those of a disease that is chronic or leaves its mark on the patient in the form of disability, or is liable to recur, or both.

Incidence means the frequency with which a specific event occurs (often a disease) within a defined population during a stated period of time. Thus, the annual incidence of new cases of a given disease, such as rheumatic fever or tuberculosis or coronary artery disease, is defined as the proportion of persons within a population who develop the disease for the first time during a given period—usually a year; correspondingly the incidence of deaths means the proportion of the population that dies in that year.

In diseases such as those just mentioned, in which recurrences of symptoms are frequently encountered, a distinction must be made between the incidence of new cases (or new patients) [2] and the incidence of multiple attacks of a disease. Since, in a given year, multiple episodes of illness may be experienced by the same individual, the latter expression gives no indication of the number of persons affected. A new case may be counted only once if the word "case" is used in its usual implication. If, on the other hand, it is the number of attacks per year that is being measured, such attacks may occur several times during this interval in a given patient.

Actually the onset of the event being measured, whether it be

[2] Medically speaking, a case is a situation of indefinite length usually involving illness in a specified individual. A patient is a person who is ill or who is under observation or who is undergoing treatment for disease.

the incidence of a disease or of acute attacks, may be insidious. Recognition of it may be delayed, either until a subsequent acute episode occurs or until other clinical evidences of a previous attack of the disease are revealed. For this reason it is sometimes necessary to consider incidence in terms of recognition rather than in terms of onset of the pathological process. Therefore, incidence rates and discovery rates could be used synonymously to express the frequency of "new cases" of a given disease.

Prevalence, on the other hand, indicates the proportion of persons in a defined population who, at a specified time, are affected or have been affected by a particular disease. Therefore, the prevalence of coronary occlusion is given as the ratio of the number of affected persons to the total population, an affected person being one who either currently has the disease or gives a history of having had one or more coronary attacks before the time of observation or shows electrocardiographic evidences thereof. Prevalence also represents the accumulated incidence of new cases during previous years from which deaths from all causes have been subtracted. A prevalence rate is further modified by those individuals with a given disease, who, prior to the time under consideration, have migrated into or out of the population.

The essential differences, therefore, between incidence and prevalence are that the latter refers to frequency at a point in time; the former to cases arising during a period of time.

Since the epidemiologist's prime duty is to make measurements of the frequency of a given disease or injury, or of deaths, one of his first activities is to determine whether the event he is about to measure is clear-cut and definite, such as an attack of measles, or indefinite, such as a disturbed mental state (perhaps too indefinite to measure). His next responsibility is to measure the size and character of the population at risk (or different groups of the population) with which he is to deal. Does the frequency differ among males and females, young and old, white and negro, rich and poor? Where and under what circumstances does the frequency of a disease differ within populations of similar and different origins that may or may not have different ways of life.

BIRTH AND DEATH RECORDS

To correlate information obtained from the census, which is calculated to throw some light on mortality as well as on related information of sanitary conditions and living conditions in the community, and on race fertility, an adequate record of births and deaths is essential. For such information, physicians, surgeons, and obstetricians have an important responsibility, although no amount of admonition here is expected to change the habits of busy doctors. Upon the accuracy and detail in which death certificates are made out depend the accuracy of age-specific and disease-specific rates to be calculated for a community. Death certificates are the very basis of information on local population pathology, that is, on the way the local killing power of certain diseases is measured. The physician's or surgeon's responsibility here is to make mortality statistics reflect the true frequencies of disease or injury in his community.

Sometimes an accurate description offers considerable difficulty that could be avoided if adequate instructions were available. In the United States, doctors can refer to the *Physician's Handbook on Death and Birth Registration* (1958), which is readily available. Furthermore, a number of lists of diagnostic terms are currently being used by hospitals in the United States. One of the best known of these is the *Standard Nomenclature of Diseases and Operations* (1961); but some institutions have recently employed a different manual for the indexing and coding of their records, namely, the *International Classification of Disease Adapted for Indexing Hospital Records by Disease and Operations* (1962). An attempt is being made to adapt this last publication for more general use in indexing hospital records in the United States. Another useful document is a leaflet, put out by the Public Health Service in 1960, entitled *Medical Certification of Causes of Death.*

Many physicians who have been devoted to the care of their patients may not consider the exact wording of the diagnosis made after the death of a patient to be of great concern either to him or to the family of the deceased. This is not true for the epidemiologically minded clinician. It is a matter of considerable concern because he must deal accurately with the diagnoses of all cases, fatal or not, in his "community" within a given time, usually with a year.

The method of listing diagnoses is also important, for the number of examples of misleading diagnoses one might quote is legion. Thus it would be an error to ascribe death to acute heart failure in a case in which the patient's heart gave out in the terminal hours of bronchial pneumonia. Some patients are found, either on clinical examination or at autopsy, to have several different kinds of lesions numerous enough to fill a shelf in a pathological museum: widespread cancer, heart disease with all its sequelae, the effects of arteriosclerosis, and terminal infection. The problem of putting one's finger on the most important illness permeates all morbidity data, and its solution calls for clinical and epidemiologic judgment. Attempts are currently being made to find suitable ways of presenting data on multiple pathological conditions existing in an individual at the time of death. In time the concept of a single cause of death may be superseded, but the difficulties of classification are formidable. Indeed, the differences in the precision and manner of labeling and the priorities ascribed to pathological syndromes may well reflect diagnostic fashions—for example, the increased popularity of coronary occlusion as a diagnostic label in death certificates (see Fig. 36). These exert some influence upon the recorded trends of disease incidence. (See Appendix 1 for some further points in making out death certificates.)

THE CRUDE DEATH RATE

The numerator is the number of deaths in a year, and the denominator is the total population within the chosen area during that year. Although this fails to take into account the age distribution of the population, it is a widely used standard. For instance, in 1949, the United States, with a population of about 150 million and 1.5 million deaths, had an annual death rate of

$$\frac{1,500,000}{150,000,000} \times 1000 = 10$$

or 10 deaths per 1,000 people. More recently in the 1960's the death rate in the United States has been about 9.3. It varies greatly in different parts of the world. In Israel it is quite low, having been recorded recently as 6.8. This is because of an unusual age distribution in that nation, which has a high percentage of young and middle-aged people.

AGE-SPECIFIC DEATH RATES

The principle is that the population is subdivided into age groups, and the number of people in each of these age groups who die during a given year is tabulated to give age-specific rates. These rates are characteristically high in infancy and old age and lowest among young adults.

DISEASE-SPECIFIC DEATH RATES

These can be estimated on a total population basis (see Fig. 9) or on an age-specific basis, the latter being much more meaningful. Coronary (ischemic) heart disease for instance, would not be considered a disease of juveniles, whereas in the 40–60 age group it becomes of great importance.

INFANT MORTALITY

An infant is defined as a child under one year of age, and the mortality in this age group is represented by the number of such infantile deaths over the number of live births in the corresponding year. This rate has special significance, since it has been used as a rough indication of local sanitary or medical standards. In 1900 in the United States, infant mortality, expressed in terms of infantile deaths per 1,000 live births, was about 100; more recently it has been recorded as around 25. In a few countries it is lower than this; in quite a number, it is much higher, ranging up to rates of 200 or more. There are a number of ways of expressing deaths which are associated with pregnancy. These appear in Appendix 1.

Some mention should be made here of standardized mortality rates, in which an attempt is made, when comparing the rates in two populations, to correct for any differences that might exist in factors such as age distribution. The primary aim is to compare the number of deaths actually observed in a given population (or among some special groups of the population) with the number expected on the basis of the age-specific death rates prevailing in other populations.

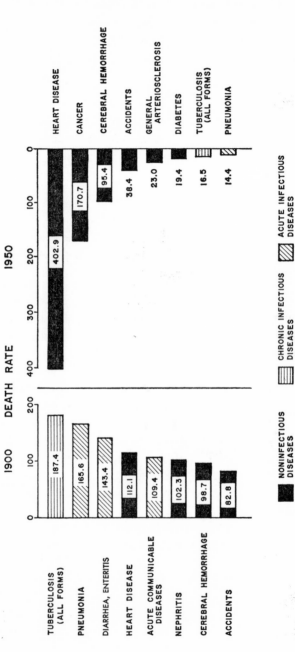

Fig. 9. Deaths per 100,000 due to eight leading causes in Connecticut in 1900 and in 1950. (Data from Keehn, R. J., 1955. Connecticut's aging population. *Conn. Health Bull.* 69:313.)

Although this preoccupation with mortality rates may seem remote from clinical epidemiology, they are emphasized because the recording of deaths is a far more accurate way of determining the frequency of certain diseases in large populations than is the recording of illnesses of various kinds, that is, the morbidity rate. The accuracy rests in part upon the definite character of the event being recorded. Doctors may argue at length whether a person is sick or not, but they rarely argue as to whether an individual is dead or not. And doctors cannot be casual about reporting a death, for it is a legal requirement in most places. Inaccuracies arise when the diagnosis at death does not reflect the true state of affairs or train of events that led to death.

On the other hand, the mortality and the morbidity of a given disease or condition obviously do not measure the same thing, and the former gives us only indirect data on the prevalence of the latter. Mortality rates, for instance, tell us very little about the importance of a variety of chronic illnesses, such as rheumatoid arthritis. If it is assumed that good medical and hospital facilities are available to all in a given community, the local death rates for cancer would be a useful index for this condition, but in the same community the death rate for measles would tell us very little about the comings and goings of that infection. Methods of determining morbidity rates will be taken up in chapter 8.

BIBLIOGRAPHY

HILL, A. BRADFORD. 1962. *Statistical methods in clinical and preventive medicine.* Edinburgh: Livingstone.

International classification of disease adapted for indexing hospital records by disease and operations. Revised, 1962. U.S. Department of Health, Education, and Welfare. Washington, D.C.: Government Printing Office.

Medical certification of causes of death. 1960. U.S. Public Service Publication No. 44. Washington, D.C.: Government Printing Office.

Physician's handbook on death and birth registration, 1958. 11th ed. U.S. Public Health Service Publication No. 593. Washington, D.C.: Government Printing Office.

Standard nomenclature of diseases and operations. 1961. 5th ed. Chicago: American Medical Association.

CHAPTER VIII

Methods and Terms
II. Illness Rates

METHODS FOR SELECTING AND LISTING CASES

Over and above the use of mortality statistics, which obviously are applicable only to certain diseases, three or four other methods have been widely used to measure the local frequency of a given disease, its incidence, prevalence, or general importance. These are: (*a*) the use of official reports from departments or ministries of health within areas or populations where certain diseases are *reportable;* (*b*) morbidity surveys, which may be set up to enumerate cases of certain diseases within a given population during a short period or for a longer period, lasting perhaps several years. The latter (so-called longitudinal surveys) are generally set up as special research projects within populations of limited size, even in a group of domiciles or a small urban or rural community, where events are carefully followed in the whole selected population. Another approach, which may be part of any survey, is (*c*) the use of local hospital or out-patient department records to determine the number of patients per year who have been admitted or discharged (or who have died) with a given diagnosis. Still another is (*d*) the so-called screening survey, using groups of normal individuals to determine past or present evidences of disease (or injury) or inapparent infection. Such surveys include: mass chest x-rays for evidence of pulmonary or mediastinal lesions; tuberculin test surveys to determine the prevalence of tuberculous infection, Shick test surveys for diphtheritic infection, and serological surveys to measure in the

78

sera of normal individuals the prevalence of certain blood components and various levels of antibodies against a variety of antigens (see chap. 9). Screening surveys are usually done on a short-term basis. In all these measurements, particularly in the screening survey, it is important to know whether the population being tested is a random or weighted sample, a matter that is taken up later in more detail in Appendix II.

An example of the significance of age can be found in the morbidity statistics of rheumatic heart disease; active rheumatic fever is essentially a disease of young people. Accordingly, incidence figures for rheumatic heart disease are often based on the number of cases detected and the calculated rate in each age group of 5–24 or 5–19 years of age. Among infants and preschool children (0–4 years) rheumatic heart disease is rare (see Fig. 10), but the commonness of congenital heart disease may be more likely to cause difficulties in diagnosis at this age.[1] At the other end of the scale among adults over 24, diagnostic difficulties also arise because combinations of cardiac lesions creep in. An analysis of heart disease rates in adults will reveal not only pure examples of inactive rheumatic heart disease, but also those in which early or advanced arteriosclerosis and other degenerative conditions are combined with or superimposed upon the old rheumatic cardiac lesion.

Statistically speaking, therefore, these are the reasons why mortality and morbidity rates for rheumatic heart disease are more useful indexes of its frequency when limited to certain age groups. This principle applies in general to all diseases characteristic of one age group, such as diseases that are common in childhood (see Fig. 10).

REPORTS FROM HEALTH DEPARTMENTS

Of the various ways of collecting morbidity statistics, the best would seem to be having a given disease officially reported (or

[1] Between the eight-year period of the writing of the first and second editions of this book, the prevalence of congenital heart conditions was recorded in the United States as having increased enormously in infants. This has been no doubt due to the success of certain surgical operations in correcting congenital cardiac conditions.

notified). Theoretically, this should be a fine method for determining either the incidence of acute attacks or the prevalence of a given disease, provided all cases are discovered, diagnosed, and conscientiously reported. The completeness with which this

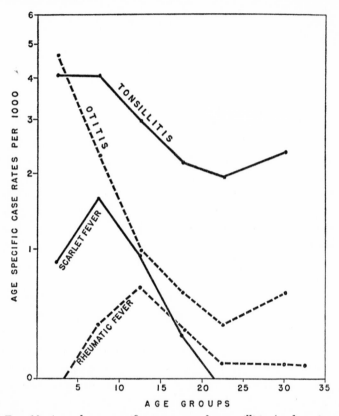

Fig. 10. Annual age-specific case rates for tonsillitis (and peritonsillar abscess), scarlet fever, otitis media, and rheumatic fever determined from white families in the eastern United States, 1928–43. The declining trends during adolescence and young adult life are evident. (Data from Collins, Trantham, and Lehman, 1955. *Sickness experience in selected areas of the United States of America.* Public Health Service Monograph No. 25.)

has been done has varied enormously, regardless of whether voluntary or compulsory reporting has been recommended, attempted, or practiced. The accuracy of local reporting was studied by Sydenstricker (1926) in the course of a sickness survey in Hagerstown, Maryland, where local physicians were aware that their "work was being checked." He found that among the reportable diseases 85 per cent of the cases of diphtheria, scarlet fever, and influenza were being reported, 60 per cent of the cases of pneumonia, 30–40 per cent of measles, pertussis, and chickenpox, and practically no cases of scabies. Interim surveys have been carried out, but, although a generation has elapsed since the original Hagerstown survey, voluntary reporting leaves much to be desired (Turner 1952).

It is understandable why certain diseases are reported more conscientiously than others and it is hard to know the accuracy of reporting which is maintained in different places or at different times. In the United States cases of smallpox or paralytic poliomyelitis, once diagnosed, would be reported with a high degree of accuracy, whereas a very large percentage of cases of pneumonia or various manifestations of streptococcal infection would go unreported. Reporting a case of syphilis, on the other hand, is a delicate matter, particularly if there is some doubt about the accuracy of the diagnosis. And there are other diseases or conditions that may be private matters, and both the patient and the physician may be loath to make them public. Under these circumstances reporting is often done by code. Some busy physicians have little enthusiasm for reporting a given disease if their efforts may only result in unfavorable publicity for their patients or in the mere gathering of statistics rather than the protection of their patients or the community. Enthusiasm may lag unless it is quite apparent why the data are being collected. The physician who is responsible for reporting should understand, nevertheless, that accurate and complete reporting of certain diseases in any community is not only desirable but indispensable in an age when infectious and noninfectious diseases are community problems as well as individual ones. More complete reporting can be expected in those places where the medical profession has been educated along these lines, and where reasons for reporting are brought to the fore and support is given to the physicians' efforts. This education is concerned not only with informing practicing physicians about disease prevalence within their community but also with how the proper authorities, if notified, can assist them, by making certain facilities, either public or private, available for the benefit of those suffering from tuberculosis, cancer, arthritis, or some of the reportable acute infectious diseases.

As a substitute for accurate reporting the establishment of a local registry has often been introduced. This has been done with tuberculosis, rheumatic fever and rheumatic heart disease, cancer of various kinds, and a number of other conditions.

MORBIDITY SURVEYS

To supplement reporting disease or injury on a national, municipal, or community scale, special surveys can be set up to find out what the local sickness experience has been. Work of this kind is being done more and more in the United States. These surveys are usually carried out on a research basis, more or less, perhaps as a university or health department project. The surveys certainly should not be engaged in lightly by groups that are not likely to be able to conduct a thorough, statistically adequate study. In the organization of these surveys questions of expense and of the required staff of clinical and statistical experts should be considered, as well as other assistants. Such surveys may be limited in time, say within a year, or they may take the form of a longitudinal survey and may cover a period of years with a staff in residence in the same community. They can utilize census tracts in a city to advantage (Foley 1953). The practicing physician may not be an active participant in this type of endeavor, but he can be of enormous assistance.

SURVEYS OF HOSPITAL RECORDS

In spite of the wide use of hospital or out-patient department records as indexes of the local prevalence of a given disease, this method is not generally recommended, particularly if the data are to be interpreted as accurate measures of local incidence. Too often these hospital data, listing the percentages of various diagnoses collected from both clinical and autopsy material, reflect the character of the hospital clientele, or local interests, or preferences of the hospital staffs, rather than a true local sampling. A prominent neurosurgeon on the staff of a given hospital may attract a large percentage of cases of brain tumors to a given clinic, so that the number of cases with this diagnosis may be given undue importance on the hospital lists. Hospital records may reflect current fashions in hospitalization, and in this respect it should be recalled that cases of pneumonia are hospitalized less often today than one decade ago. On the other hand, the method does have its uses, and a very valuable and extensive series of prevalence figures have been assembled by Fraenkel and Erhardt (1955) from the municipal hospitals of New York City.

SCREENING SURVEYS

Screening surveys are those that attempt to make quick reviews of illness within a given population, presumably by examinations and tests easily performed to be carried out within a few days or weeks. The information derived from such surveys often suffers because those who present themselves for the required tests are not randomly selected but are volunteers—particularly those enterprising volunteers interested in obtaining a free medical opinion. This may give rise to a highly weighted group. Obviously the result depends on the random character of the sampling methods used, the nature of any physical examination or tests (x-rays, blood sugar and urine, blood lipids, and various serologic tests), the accuracy with which the specimens are handled and the tests performed, and a number of other features that can easily go wrong. The approach represents a whole subject in itself and some of it will be discussed in the chapter on serologic epidemiology and in Appendix 2.

SURVEY TECHNIQUES THE PHYSICIAN CAN USE

The epidemiologist's prime duty is to make measurements of the frequency of a given disease or injury, or death in defined populations in a designated area—in a family living on a farm, in a tenement house, in a new housing project, or in a larger population. Where and under what circumstances does this

83

disease seem to be most frequent; where most rare? Are differences in prevalence apparent within kindreds, in ethnic groups, in various occupations, in groups with different diets or ways of life? The frequency of the disease in question is fundamental. The likelihood of tracking down uncommon diseases or conditions is not particularly hopeful unless there is a large population. With a common disease one can be more hopeful.

APARTMENT-HOUSE EXAMPLE

To illustrate what is meant here and what an analysis of these measurements might mean, let us imagine a situation in which the incidence of acute attacks of seasonal bronchial asthma differed appreciably among people living in one part of an apartment house than in another. The difference in incidence could be due to a variety of circumstances. The first task would be to determine the number of occupants of the apartment house, as much information about their age, sex, and background as one could conveniently accumulate, and then as much information about the site as possible. If the observations were made during the late summer or ragweed season, it might be found that a ragweed patch was located to the north of the apartment house and that the prevailing wind was from the north. Conceivably this could explain a heavier incidence of attacks among the inhabitants of those apartments on the north side of the building.

On the other hand, the effect could be reversed, if the occupants of the northern half lived and slept with their windows closed all day and night while those in the southern half kept theirs open. Or it might happen that the entire eastern half of the apartment house was occupied by a large group of blood relatives, among whom there was a hereditary tendency to allergic conditions. In this instance, there might be an increase well above the expected rate in the incidence of attacks of bronchial asthma among residents of the eastern half of the apartment house population as compared with those of the western. Such an increase would not, under these circumstances, mean that there was more ragweed pollen floating about in the air around the eastern half of the apartment house, but that there was a greater number of susceptible hosts. Thus, bit by bit, circumstances explaining the different incidences of attack rates could be brought to light by the proper investigation, the proper choice of questions to be asked, and the proper choice of measurements.

METHODOLOGY OF COUNTING CASES

Few of the various recognized ways for determining the incidence or prevalence of some of our most important diseases are thoroughly satisfactory. Theoretically the simplest method of determining the incidence or prevalence or distribution of a given disease is to look at the reports available in a given health department to see how many people are listed as living within the department's jurisdiction, their ages, sex, marital status, and race, and the number who died or were sick from that disease in a given year. Such data are available in many parts of the world. But if incidence data are derived from municipal or state morbidity statistics, certain common diseases will usually be found to suffer from underreporting, such as tuberculosis, rheumatic fever, coronary occlusion, and, of course, cancer.

First comes the question of having reasonably accurate figures for our ratio, n/P, where n equals the number of cases (or deaths) that occur within a given time, and P equals the size of the population at risk. For our purpose, P (the community) may be very small, indeed no larger than a single household. But most problems in epidemiology deal with a larger community and require population data from a regular system of census-taking to obtain the essential denominator. In the United States the census is taken every ten years, and for interim years an estimation on the basis of previous population trends is usually made. The mere counting of heads is not enough, however, for adequate comparisons of mortality or morbidity experience cannot be made between any two or more districts or populations without information relating to the ages and sexes of the people comprising the communities. Such information is not likely to be available, in many out-of-the-way places. Here the epidemiologist will have to make certain compromises when limited by the lack of vital statistics.

It will not be our function here to indicate how censuses should be taken but merely to mention how essential they are to the epidemiologist and how certain ancillary types of information are desirable. This includes the limitation of the data to a single unit of time; the division into geographical areas, particularly those which concern rural and urban ways of living; and the division of the population into age groups, including infants, 0–1 year of age, preschool children, 1–4, and other groups 5–9, 10–14, 15–19, 20–24, 25–34, 35–44, and so on. Other data are concerned with the distribution of the sexes; racial designations, particularly those of white and non-white groups, occupation and socioeconomic status.

BIBLIOGRAPHY

COLLINS, S. D., TRANTHAM, K. S., and LEHMANN, J. L. 1954. Sickness experience in selected areas of the United States. Monograph 25. Washington, D.C.: Department of Health, Education, and Welfare, Public Health Service.

FOLEY, D. L. 1953. Census tracts and urban research. *J. Am. Statistical Assoc.* 48:733–42.

FRAENKEL, M. and ERHARDT, C. L. 1955. *Morbidity in the municipal hospitals of the City of New York*. New York: Russell Sage Foundation.

National Health Survey. 1957. *U.S. Public Health Service. Public Health Rept.* 75:5–8.

National Health Survey Act. Public Law 652, 1956. 84th Congress, 2d session. Washington, D.C.: U.S. Government Printing Office.

SYDENSTRICKER, E. 1926a. A study of illness in a general population. Hagerstown Morbidity studies, No. 1. *Public Health Rept.* 41:2069.

———. 1926b. The reporting of notifiable diseases in a typical small city. *Public Health Rept.* 41:2186.

TURNER, V. B. 1952. *Hagerstown health studies and annotated bibliography.* Public Health Bibliography Ser. No. 6 (Publication 148). Washington, D.C.: Department of Health, Education, and Welfare, Public Health Service.

World Health Organization. 1957. *Expert committees on health statistics. Fifth Rept. Tech. Rept. Series, 133.* Geneva.

Methods and Terms
III. Charting Data

CHARTING CASES

Many individuals gain more information from the visual impact of a situation expressed in the form of an equation than from a diagram, regardless whether the event depicted is an epidemiological one or not. For the use of equations to express epidemics or the use of statistics in epidemiology in general one can refer to various texts, particularly to the one by Bradford Hill (1961), and to the one dealing more with the theoretical aspects by Moench (1959), and no doubt to scores of others that I should be ill-qualified to discuss. I shall limit myself in this chapter to graphic methods and the use of simple diagrams.

One of the simplest and easiest ways of charting or depicting a series of illnesses that have occurred within a community is to mark the onset of each case on a calendar scale with some kind of legend and thus illustrate temporal relationships between individual cases.[1] One can start with a group as small as a family and indicate on a chart what happens during the course of an infection. Figure 11 shows that an unknown amount of the infecting agent, hemolytic streptococci, was introduced into the family group at some time prior to January 1, which was the day of onset of the first clinical cases of streptococcal infection. This is an acute type of infection usually spread via the respiratory tract between individuals within a setting characteristic of the

---

[1] The onset of many diseases has been designated as the first day of illlness. This may differ, of course, from the day of recognition.

association which family life entails. From a glance at events that took place in this family, one can see that five cases appeared in

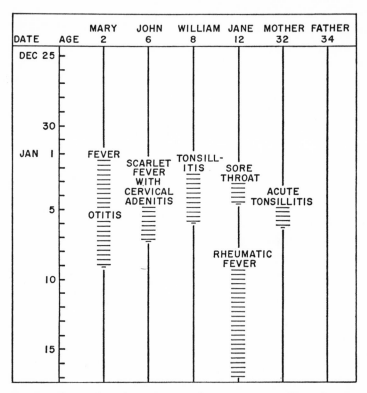

FIG. 11. This epidemiologic diagram designates six members of a given family and what happened to them during a 15-day period in January. These family members are portrayed by a series of vertical lines, with their names and ages at the top. The scale of time is shown at the left, covering a period of three weeks. Streptococcal infections within the family, which began more or less simultaneously, are indicated by a series of short horizontal lines. In four of the five members who were ill, the disease expressed itself in a slightly different form, perhaps reflecting the age and degree of "immunological maturity" of the person infected. (From J. R. Paul [ed.], 1943. *The epidemiology of rheumatic fever and some of its public health aspects.* 2d ed. New York: Metropolitan Life Insurance Co.)

the first week of January. From this concentration, it is fair to assume that most of the cases were exposed more or less simultaneously; but whether all these exposures were actually derived from a common extra-domiciliary source (for instance, contaminated milk) or whether the infection was brought into the family by one member and passed rapidly to other members is not evident from the chart because the incubation in this infection is so short (one to four days).[2] Nevertheless, this was an explosive family epidemic, especially from the viewpoint of the mother of the family, for when the whole family becomes sick at one time, she is burdened by an "outburst" of new (and unwanted) responsibilities. The infection in this particular instance expressed itself in different clinical forms, such as sore throat with fever terminating with otitis, scarlet fever, and acute tonsillitis. In one instance, the acute infection was followed by the complication of rheumatic fever (Paul 1943). There is a relationship between age and various clinical forms of acute streptococcal infection and as this family was made up, as most families are, of individuals of different ages here is a situation involving differing degrees of host susceptibility—a subject to be discussed later.

It is only a step to extend the type of chart indicated in Fig. 11 from the family to a small or large community. The chart marking the onset of individual cases can also be drawn on a calendar scale. A classic example of a milk-borne epidemic of streptococcal infection is shown in Fig. 12. The epidemic was described a generation ago in Denmark, where records of diseases have been kept with more accuracy and for a longer period of time than in most countries (Madsen and Kalbak 1940). There was a concentration of cases of streptococcal infection in which many of the onsets occurred within a short (seven-day) period, suggesting the simultaneous exposure of many people to the milk that, in this instance, was contaminated with *Streptococcus hemolyticus*. The curve, which rises rapidly to a peak and then declines slowly, would make one suspect that in the last week in November there had been a sudden and widespread introduction of this infectious agent in heavy dos-

[2] An *incubation period* of an infectious disease means the period of time between that of entrance of the infectious agent into the body and the onset of the symptoms of the consequent disease.

ages into the community; there was less evidence of this during the next three weeks.[3] This suspicion might not have been warranted had the curve been gradual and more like a mountain range or a plateau.

The secondary epidemic of rheumatic fever, beginning on December 19 (see Fig. 12), indicates the proportion that became

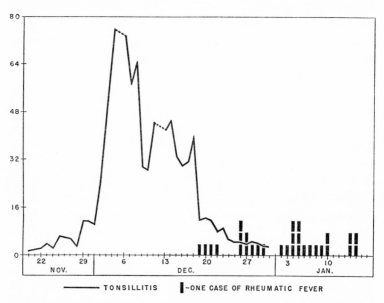

Fɪɢ. 12. Severe milk-borne epidemic of hemolytic streptococcal infection that occurred in Denmark in 1926 and was associated with or followed by an "epidemic" of rheumatic fever. The scale on the left indicates the daily number of cases of tonsillitis, so-called septic sore throat. Late in the epidemic, 30 cases of rheumatic fever appeared. (From Madsen and Kalbak, 1940. *Acta. Pathol. Microbiol. Scand.* **17**:305.)

infected with Group A streptococcus, (often quoted as 3 per cent), whose streptoccal infection may or not have been overt, and yet who developed rheumatic fever as a sequela. For a number of understandable reasons this latter group of cases is

[3] The dose of streptococci present in a glass of milk may be sufficient to produce disease in a high percentage of those who drink the milk. But these infected milk-drinkers may be incapable of putting out streptococci in large enough quantities to infect their associates to the same degree.

less concentrated in point of time, but it could be designated as an epidemic. Here the "incubation" or latent period is longer (ten to twenty days); it varies more, and therefore the grouping of cases covers a wider spread.

The demonstration of the "explosive" epidemic, in a disease with a short incubation period and its capacity to form a characteristic peaklike curve, suggesting a sudden dose of infecting organisms from a common source, may be an oversimplification in that it disregards certain important factors that tend to prolong or stop epidemics. First comes the question of whether there was opportunity for the etiologic agent to spread further in the population, beyond those who were originally infected from drinking milk or from another common source. If so, a train of events could be touched off, to be reflected by a series of subsequent waves in the epidemic curve, and the original peak is blotted out. Next, the hypothetical development of "acute" immunity in the exposed and inapparently infected members of the population might proceed so rapidly that the supply of susceptibles in the population would be soon used up, and correspondingly the epidemic might burn itself out in short order. This would be true particularly if the population were small. Third, an influx of new susceptibles into the population at risk might prolong the epidemic. These and other factors are to be considered before an attempt to interpret the epidemic curve is made. Other factors to be considered include the length of the incubation period, the size of the dose of the infectious agent, its source, and the method of spread.

With a disease like measles, for instance, which is a viral infection spread through human association (by contact, as some have called it), the opportunities for its spread are many, provided there are local susceptible hosts available. The incubation period is about two weeks, however, and the period when the patient transmits the disease is brief and limited to the onset of his illness. As a result, when this virus is introduced into a single family or multiple families or households, one may see a primary wave representing the initial cases, which infects the other exposed members in turn, and this gives rise to a secondary wave two weeks later, and perhaps a tertiary wave. When, on the other hand, the incubation period of a given disease is longer than three weeks, the variability of this period may yield misleading interpretations of the epidemiological curve as to whether a common source or multiple sources of infection are responsible.

A special example of the latter situation was the outbreak of serum hepatitis among United States Army troops during World War II (Parr 1945). This unfortunate accident was the result of the inoculation of troops with yellow fever vaccine in which human serum had been used as a stabilizing agent. Certain batches of the serum contained serum hepatitis virus (so-called hepatitis virus B, or virus SH). Serum hepatitis not only has a long incubation period ranging from fifty to two hundred days, but there are great variations in its length. Consequently, although a common-source outbreak of postvaccinal cases of hepatitis, when charted, could yield a skyscraper-like curve, the chances are it would not. A situation of this kind was studied by Parr in a military outbreak of serum hepatitis that occurred in 1942 at Camp Polk, Louisiana, where, as the result of inoculations of an icterogenic lot of yellow fever vaccine, an epidemic of 1,004 cases of serum hepatitis resulted (see Fig. 13). These cases occurred only in vaccinees, all of whom had received the same dose of vaccine, all on the same day. The variability in length of the incubation periods ranged from 60 to 160 days **giving the** appearance of a prolonged epidemic in which the infection was passed along from man to man. If the cause of this situation had not eventually become known, the medical officers in charge would not have realized that the infection was actually due to a common source. It would be unwise to say today with complete assurance that a few of the cases illustrated in Fig. 13 might not have resulted from secondary infection (transmission through association or contact), but this is not supposed to take place with serum hepatitis and, therefore, is unlikely.

There are a great variety of examples of epidemiological charts that seek to portray graphically a series of cases at a point in time within a population. There is no routine way of setting down in regulated fashion the welter of information that the function of recording multiple infections, particularly, entails. Within the past two decades, the task has grown more complicated because the number of new enteroviruses and respiratory viruses have increased mightily. The variability of symptoms that these viruses have produced covers a wide spectrum (Horstmann 1965), and of course many of these are silent infections that do not give rise to any symptoms at all. Thus any chart which

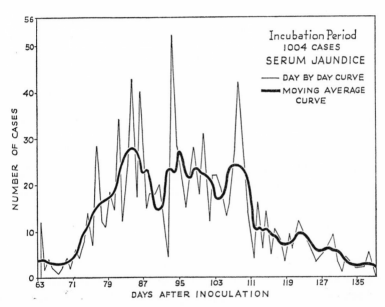

FIG. 13. Prolonged outbreak of serum hepatitis for which variations in the incubation period were responsible. The epidemic took place in a military camp among 1,004 men inoculated simultaneously with the same dose of the same lot of vaccine. (Data from Parr, 1945. *Med. Ann. District Columbia* **14**:443.)

attempts to give a picture of the whole story or impact of such infections within an institutional population is an ambitious task. It would have to portray the number and variety of illnesses, the time of their appearance, and the time of appearance of the infectious agents. The identification of the serum antibodies to any of the suspected causal infectious agents (viral or bacterial) should be recorded on matched serum samples, if possible. It is easy to see that such a task would require a large team of clinical investigators, microbiologists, and other assistants, not to mention the almost mandatory services of a computer. Consequently one should be left to one's own devices to choose the kind or kinds of charts supported by data in tabular form that will allow the most information to be packed into the diagram without being too confusing. For one rule about charts is, that, if graphic illustrations are to be used, they should illustrate.

THE SPOT MAP

Another familiar technique in charting epidemiological data is that of marking the geographical sites where various cases of a given disease or injury arose, that is, the spot map. Occasionally this can be of value in locating the cause of the trouble. This method of portraying the distribution of disease dates back to the eighteenth century (Stevenson 1965), and perhaps before. Early and classic examples were maps of the yellow fever epidemics in Philadelphia in the 1790's and John Snow's map of the Broad Street pump in London in the mid-nineteenth century, to which reference was made in an earlier chapter. His dots, indicating cases of cholera, on a map of one section of the city revealed a concentration of such cases about one of the local water supplies. The distribution of dots about the Broad Street pump was an indication that those who lived in its immediate vicinity were more likely to be stricken with cholera than those who did not; it was but a simple matter of house-to-house questioning to establish whether the patients (or the deceased) had actually used the pump, the inference being that the water from the pump was contaminated.[4] The historic interpretation of this episode was based upon a number of assumptions. First, one assumes a common denominator in population density available for the various sections of London; in other words, for the

---

[4] This type of house-to-house epidemiological survey involves the expenditure of considerable time and energy and requires a certain amount of detective work, but it can sometimes be a most rewarding form of practical epidemiology. It has the humble name of "shoe-leather epidemiology."

concentration of cases to mean what a quick glance at the map implies, one assumes that the population density in the area around the pump was about the same as that of surrounding districts. In this instance there was little reason to suspect otherwise. Next, one must assume that the same homogeneity existed with regard to resistance or susceptibility to this infection throughout the population. Here again, one need not suspect differences in London in the mid-nineteenth century. And finally, one has to assume that the great majority, if not all, of the cases spotted on the map were actually water-borne and not spread by other means, such as association with an active human carrier of cholera vibrios who might by chance be living in the area of the pump. In the event of the latter contingency, the concentration of water-borne cases about the pump might soon be blotted out. The incrimination of the Broad Street pump was established when Snow actually visited these homes and questioned members of each household about their drinking water. Also the well was inspected and found defective; and, as a simple preventive measure, the pump handle was removed.

To illustrate how on occasion the spot map may require special interpretation and why its use is only one of the clinical epidemiologist's leads, one may quote another example. In a large eastern city a number of cases of murine typhus suddenly appeared more or less simultaneously, and the local epidemiologist immediately set himself to the task of spotting the cases on a map. This rickettsial disease is spread through the agency of a rat flea. Because of this mode of spread, its incidence has been demonstrated to be greater among persons whose home or whose work brings them in contact with places to which rats are attracted, such as places for storing groceries, granaries, and refuse dumps. In the situation mentioned here, the homes of the cases were charted, revealing a scattered distribution throughout the city. Not until the sites where these patients worked were charted on the map did a concentration of cases become apparent. The railroad station, where food was unloaded and stored, was the source of contamination (Maxcy 1926).

Another pitfall ever-present in the use of the spot map can be illustrated by the instance of a small outbreak of poliomyelitis that occurred in a summer camp for boys in New England in the 1930's. In a camp population totaling about one hundred boys, who ranged in age from eleven to eighteen, four cases of recognized poliomyelitis occurred within a period of five days. This called for an immediate consultation and investigation. The boys had been quartered in a group of eleven cabins arranged in the shape of a U, with about nine boys in each cabin. The four cases were in Cabins 1, 2, and 3, as illustrated in Fig. 14.

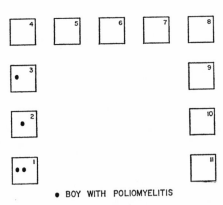

Fig. 14. Spot map of the arrangement of cabins at a boys' camp where four cases of poliomyelitis occurred within a few days of one another. Each cabin housed approximately nine boys. The boys became progressively older as one moved around the U from left to right so that the concentration of cases on the left does not necessarily imply that location was the only factor. An increase of age-susceptibility seems much more likely. (From unpublished data collected in 1939 by the Yale Poliomyelitis Study Unit.)

Although it might seem that some special and localized source of exposure to poliomyelitis virus could have been responsible for the concentration of cases, a more likely explanation was that the degree of exposure had been the same for all boys, but, since the youngest boys lived in the cabins shown in the lower left-hand corner of the diagram, the boys being progressively older as one moved around the U, there was an unequal distribution of age susceptibility in the camp population. This is based on the principle that the degree of resistance to frank poliomyelitis rose gradually with age, a fact which was more apparent in the 1930's prior to the use of prophylactic vaccination against poliomyelitis.

BIBLIOGRAPHY

HILL, A. BRADFORD. 1961. *Principles of medical statistics.* 7th ed. New York: Oxford University Press.

HORSTMANN, D. M. 1965. Clinical Virology. *Am. J. Med.* 38:738–49.

MADSEN, T. and KALBAK, N. 1940. Investigations on rheumatic fever subsequent to epidemics of septic sore throat (especially milk epidemics). *Acta. Pathol. Microbiol. Scand.* 17:305.

MAXCY, K. F. 1926. An epidemiological study of endemic typhus (Brill's disease) in the southeastern United States, with special reference to its mode of transmission. *Public Health Rept.* 41:1.

MUENCH, HUGO. 1959. *Catalytic models in epidemiology.* Cambridge, Mass.: Harvard University Press.

PARR, L. W. 1945. Host variations in the manifestation of disease with particular reference to homologous serum jaundice in the Army of the United States. *Med. Ann. District of Columbia* 14:443.

PAUL, J. R. (ed.) 1943. *The epidemiology of rheumatic fever and some of its public health aspects.* 2d ed. New York: Metropolitan Life Insurance Co.

STEVENSON, L. G. 1965. Putting disease on the map. The early use of spot maps in the study of yellow fever. *J. Hist. Med.* 20:226–61.

CHAPTER X

Population Information

As people represent the material upon which our subject of epidemiology is based, it will be the purpose of this chapter to deal with demography, or population studies, from the standpoint of health (Dunn 1956, Rogers 1960).[1] But an apology is necessary, for, as demography is an extensive and special subject in itself and reflects a changing scene within the United States and elsewhere, its treatment here will have to be brief, somewhat superficial, and in many ways inadequate.

It is to the current census and to the local health department and its division of vital statistics that most physicians turn for their information about populations, health conditions, and trends of disease within their local communities and cities. For instance, one can usually determine, in the United States at least, the total number of people living within a given area according to the last census, their ages, sexes (see Fig. 16), and the relative racial percentages. Added to this it is obviously desirable to know the local birth and death rates, and particularly the current and past frequency with which reportable and even some nonreportable diseases, illnesses, or accidents have occurred. Other features desirable to know are: the local seasonal effect upon the rates for diseases and injury; what areas in the community are prone to high rates of this or that illness; and what the impact of local industrial practices or living conditions

---

[1] For a review of population information I particularly recommend Part I (Demographic Background) of the text by E. S. Rogers, *Human Ecology and Health* (New York: Macmillan Co. 1960), pp. 1–100.

is upon this picture. It is obvious that, if one is to understand or interpret these data, one must know the people from whom they come, for diseases shift constantly, with growth or decline of populations, changing customs, new fashions, and new ways of living.

GROWTH OF POPULATIONS

In most parts of the world the size of the population is far from static. Since 1900 the population of the United States had doubled from 76 million to 151 million in 1950. It had reached 180 million by 1960. At least three factors are operating here at a given time: the birth rate, the migration rate, and the death rate. All of them can fluctuate, sometimes suddenly. During the 1920's the birth rate in the United States showed a steady decline, and it was believed that low birth rates would be a characteristic trend of the American population. Thus the birth rate had dropped from more than 30 per 1,000 population in 1900 to less than 19 in the depression years of the 1930's. But with the beginning of reemployment, a subsequent boom in war industries and probably a number of other factors, this trend was sharply reversed, and by 1950 the United States birth rate averaged around 25 per 1,000. It has remained at about this level for more than a decade but recently has declined slightly.

Another factor which may contribute to the growth of a population is immigration from abroad. This has not played an important part since the early 1920's in the United States but may again soon as a result of proposed changes in immigration restrictions. Furthermore, within the nation, intracontinental migration has given rise to a disproportionate regional growth in some areas, such as southern California, and has contributed much to an increase in some urban populations. The ever-increasing world population, the so-called "population explosion" needs no elaboration here, but this is not to imply that we do not recognize its seriousness, or that we know how it is to be dealt with.

99

DEATH RATES

The decline in the total death (crude mortality) rate [2] in the United States has had a marked effect upon the total population as well as upon its age composition. To say that this has been a prominent trend in the United States during the past half-century is an understatement (see Fig. 15). This fall in death rates has been due to many factors, prominent among which has

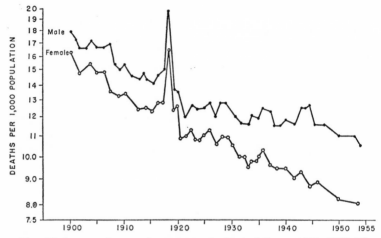

FIG. 15. Sex-specific mortality rates in the United States, 1900–1954. The male rates have declined more slowly than the female. (Data from The Health Information Foundation, New York, 1956. 4: No. 1.)

been the curtailment of mortality risks in both young and old from infectious diseases such as pneumonia, streptococcal illnesses, even tuberculosis. Not all this lengthening of the life span has come to pass under the aegis of the medical profession or of public health administrators, or so-called public health educators. Building contractors, who are usually quick to recognize

[2] Definitions may be in order here. The crude mortality rate is the number of deaths recorded during a calendar year per 1,000 people in the total population. Age-adjusted mortality rates represent rates adjusted to allow for changes in the age distribution within the population. Refinements in the measurement of mortality, usually designated as sex-specific, age-specific, cause-specific, or combinations of these, are often used. For other definitions, see chapter 7.

that comfort and longevity are desirable commodities, as well as plumbers and manufacturers of refrigerators have all had their share in reducing the hazards of life due to acute illness. Today urban American living calls for surroundings that would seem very artificial to our great-grandparents, or even our grandparents. Nevertheless the labor saving devices and the lack of consistent physical activity may not be the blessings they might seem to be, particularly for the male who does not seem as tolerant of an office- or desk-bound existence as the female.

At the turn of the century death rates were high in the United States although they soon began to decline, the rates for females being about the same as that for the males (see Fig. 15). In the 1930's, however, which was a time when infectious disease began to become much less important (see Fig. 18), a noticeable change began to occur. The female death rate continued its decline at about the same speed, but the male rate showed less tendency to decline. No doubt coronary heart disease which is such an important cause of death in the middle-aged male contributed to this, but in any event the U.S. population has more women than men in the older age brackets as of 1960 (see Fig. 16).

INCREASING LIFE EXPECTANCY

Children born in the United States in the 1940's could look forward to an average of nearly seventy years of life, whereas at the turn of the century they were expected to live, on the average, only forty-seven years.[3] This reflects the national story of the decline in death rates, which has not taken place at the same speed within all segments of the population. The value of considering the changes happening in our population lies not so much in showing the average length of life a group of babies

---

[3] This concept of life expectancy is computed on the assumption that, as a group of newborn infants goes through life, its members will experience the age-specific mortality rates that prevailed the year that they were born. Or to put it another way, life expectancy at birth tells us how long a group of babies will live, on the average, if the mortality patterns existing at time of birth remain constant throughout their life span.

may expect, but rather in summarizing the total mortality picture of a particular population group at a given point in time. How much this may differ in different parts of the world can be seen from a glance at Fig. 17, which deals with the variation in life expectancy at birth for a number of selected countries, as computed fairly recently (1946 to 1952). In India for the years

POPULATION PYRAMID OF THE UNITED STATES IN 1960

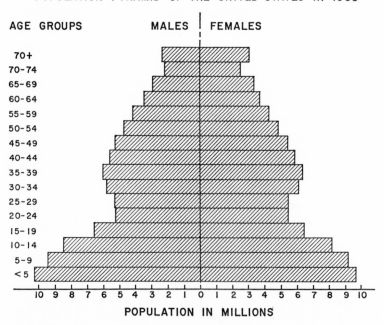

FIG. 16. Data from United States Bureau of the Census, 1960.

1941 to 1950 the life expectancy of males at birth was only thirty-two years. At the other extreme, females born in Norway from 1946 to 1950 had an average life expectancy of seventy-three years.

The United States occupies a position in the lower half of this chart. Its population, widely dispersed over a large land area, is made up of many diverse elements and subgroups with various economic and educational patterns. An example of this can be found in the differences between white and Negro; consistently

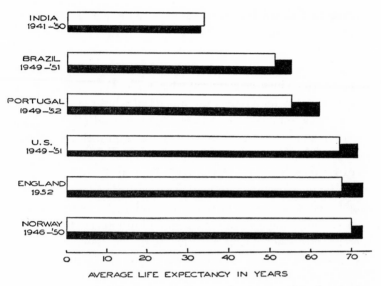

Fig. 17. Life expectancy at birth, by sex, for certain selected countries. The black horizontal columns represent the female; the white, the male. (Data from The Health Information Foundation, New York, 1956. 4: No. 4.)

the white population has a longer life expectancy than the Negro.

INFANT MORTALITY

Another and most important aspect of this situation is infant mortality which, besides affecting the total population and its age composition, is considered to be one of the more apparent indications of the sanitary status of a community, at least by Western standards. Infant mortality rates, measured by the number of babies who die before they reach their first birthday, per 1,000 live births, have dropped in the United States from nearly 100 in 1915 to 26 in 1960. The slope of the decline has been greater for Negro babies than for white. Considerable differences now exist within the fifty states of the Union, and theoretically corrections should be made for the various ratios within each state for white and Negro; in 1952 the overall extremes of infant mortality in the United States ranged from 20.7 to 47.5.

103

Over and above the fact that the infant mortality rate has earned the reputation of being a sensitive index of health conditions, particularly of diarrheal diseases, this rate has on occasion an indirect bearing upon the frequency of other diseases which may be acquired later in life. For instance, a high infant mortality may reflect the impact of wholesale exposure in infancy to a number of infections, intestinal and otherwise, and from this exposure infants either may die from such infections or emerge with more immunity than exists among those who are not so exposed early in life (Payne 1955, Paul 1958). In like manner, a low infant mortality rate may reflect a low exposure rate that might well result in an increase of childhood or adolescent ill-nesses, which might have been acquired in infancy, but are now merely postponed. Coincidently, with an improvement in infant mortality there is apt to be a general improvement in health administration, including an improvement in the way diseases, vital statistics, and so on are recorded. Such an improvement may seem to have brought about an increase in the numbers of recognized illnesses, but this might be attributable to the underreporting that had gone on in the past. The latter feature has not been evaluated.

CHANGING AGE COMPOSITION OF POPULATIONS

At any given time the size of a given population, its age composition, and its vulnerability to a variety of diseases is

TABLE 1

PERCENTAGE DISTRIBUTION OF UNITED STATES POPULATION BY AGE
(1900–1955)

Age Groups	1900	1920	1950	1960
0–19 years.........	44.3	38.8	33.9	38.5
20–44 years.........	33.7	38.3	37.6	32.3
45–64 years.........	13.7	17.5	20.3	20.2
65–85 + years	4.4	5.6	8.2	9.2

Data from *1960 United States Census of Population, U.S. Summary* (1962 and *Current Population Reports, Population Estimates* (Washington, D.C.: U.S. Department of Commerce and Bureau of the Census).

reflected, as previously stated, by the birth rate, the death rate, and increments to the population from immigration. In the

United States the declining birth and death rates, along with heavy immigration during the first two decades of the twentieth century, resulted in 1960, not only in an increase in the total population but in an increased percentage of older people (see Table 1). It is hardly necessary to take time to point out how this aging or aged population would affect the character of employment, customs and ways of living, the increasing use of apartments as dwellings, migration to the warmer parts of the country, and most importantly, the character and frequency of diseases prone to attack such a population.

CHANGES IN THE LEADING CAUSES OF DEATH

CURTAILMENT OF INFECTIOUS DISEASE

During the past fifty years a remarkable degree of control, both prophylactic and therapeutic, has been developed over many of the most important communicable (infectious) diseases —pneumonia, streptococcal infections, tuberculosis, some enteric infections, and the virus diseases of poliomyelitis and measles. Thus the current death rate for influenza and pneumonia per 100,000 population has dropped since 1900 from 202 to 34; for tuberculosis from 194 to 27; and the rate for diphtheria has fallen from 40 to less than 1.

Particularly prominent has been the declining rate of certain enteric infections, of which typhoid fever is a notable example. This also reflects to some degree the standard of sanitation in the local environment; high rates for typhoid fever, for instance, have long been regarded as a black mark on the service record of the health officer. To a lesser extent, rates for acute infectious diseases, many of which are preventable today, represent a similar index, and the speed with which they have declined in many countries during the past fifty years is impressive. Figure 18 shows the experience of the United States. Among the ten leading causes of death in 1900, the communicable diseases accounted for 36 per cent of the total deaths in the United States. Today they account for only 5 per cent of all deaths.

What is happening in one section of the country and how the

relative incidence of certain diseases are wont to change has been illustrated earlier (see Fig. 9). Changes in the type and the rates of fatal diseases in the state of Connecticut during the past half-century are illustrated in two columns giving the eight leading causes of death in 1900 compared with 1950. Obviously these causes of death will vary enormously in different parts of the world and also within different segments of the population of the same general area.

INCREASE IN NONINFECTIOUS DISEASE

Today in the United States, chronic illness and disability have replaced acute infectious diseases. Since many of these diseases

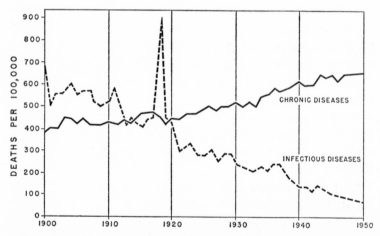

FIG. 18. Deaths per 100,000 population from chronic diseases and from acute infectious diseases in the United States, 1900–1950. (From *Building America's health: A report to the President by the President's Commission on the health needs of the nation.* Washington: Government Printing Office, 1952. Basic data from the National Office of Vital Statistics.)

are obscure in origin and slow in development, the diagnosis often lags and knowledge of their frequency and epidemiology has not gone forward as fast as one might like. New methods of measuring the occurrence and the severity of chronic disease are greatly needed, as well as more knowledge about the relationships that the frequency of one disease bears to another.

In this connection the charts measuring death rates (see Fig. 9, 15, and 17) are not necessarily measures of the total good or bad health in the community. Nevertheless, for reasons already discussed, epidemiological analyses must necessarily rely on death rates as indices of what is happening in the community, although, since death is inevitable, it is only the premature death that can be regarded as a measure of health deficiency. As a number of communicable diseases are, by and large, diseases that afflict young people, any reduction of fatal cases due to such diseases should have a very appreciable effect upon the age composition of the surviving population, increasing the percentage of older people. Thus one finds many more people in the total population today who are able to acquire the "diseases of old age," such as cardiovascular renal disease or cancer. To some extent the improvements in the picture of diseases of early life are responsible for this, and, as a consequence, we again come to a concept that every disease is indirectly related, as far as its prevalence is concerned, with every other disease. Therefore, it is clear that although age-specific case rates for senile diseases may not have changed markedly within recent decades, the vastly increased significance today of chronic disease is due largely to the increased number of people in the older age brackets, who are both susceptible and available subjects for chronic disease. Thus today chronic diseases have found a better place for themselves, so to speak, because of shifts in the age composition of the population that are taking place in many countries. The picture in the United States is a reminder of this familiar fact (see Table 1).

BIBLIOGRAPHY

Building America's Health: A Report to the President by the President's Commission on the Health Needs of the Nation. 1952. Washington, D.C.: Government Printing Office.

DUNN, H. L. 1956. *Health and demography.* Washington, D.C.: Department of Health, Education, and Welfare, Office of Vital Statistics.

PAUL, J. R. 1958. Infantile mortality rates and poliomyelitis. An epidemiological study. *Science* 127:1062.

PAYNE, A. M.-M. 1955. Poliomyelitis as a world problem. In *Papers and discussions at the 3d international poliomyelitis conference.* Philadelphia: J. B. Lippincott Co.

Progress in health services. 1956–57. Vol. IV. New York: Health Information Foundation.

ROGERS, E. S. 1960. *Human ecology and health.* New York: Macmillan Co.

Statistical abstract of the United States. 1963. 84th ed. Publication 1036. Prepared under the direction of EDWIN D. GOLDFIELD. United States Department of Commerce, Washington, D.C.: Government Printing Office.

CHAPTER XI

Host Susceptibility in Man

In a previous chapter it was pointed out that it is generally easier to measure experimentally the dosage of a poison, or a drug, or a bacterium than it is to measure the host's resistance to these agents. Nevertheless, measurements of host resistance take up the epidemiologist's time with an ever increasing variety of tests and their analyses. The significance of these studies has already been partially discussed but only from the experimental standpoint and for the most part in mice. In the present chapter we will be concerned with susceptibility or resistance in man. What are the known, measurable features that make some people more vulnerable or resistant to illness or injury than others? To what extent is this vulnerability due to genetic features? To what extent has it been acquired through exposure to disease or through training to withstand it or, in the case of an infectious disease, through immunity?

THE IMPACT OF HUMAN GENETICS ON EPIDEMIOLOGY

Increasing realization of the importance of genetics to medicine has led to the establishment of courses in this subject, even departments in many medical schools. Practicing physicians, clinical investigators, and public health workers, in fact all those who use epidemiological techniques have to be aware that man is genetically heterogenous. Thus understanding the nature of the inborn genetic diversity of human beings is an essential prerequisite for the epidemiologist. The difficulties revolve mainly around the old problem of understanding what is meant by the phenotype and how to distinguish it from the genotype.[1] The term "phenotype" describes the human subject as representative of an organism upon whom the environment has had its effect, whereas the term "genotype" refers to a much more hypothetical concept of the human organism prior to any impact of the environment.

Man's physical and mental make-up stems from a multiplicity of convergent factors. Except for identical twins no human beings have identical genes, and no two persons are exposed to the same environment. Genes contain the information encoded in their chemical structure that is translated into the developmental pattern of the individual in his embryonic, juvenile, and adult life. Although the science of genetics has been developing since the days of Gregor Mendel, a large measure of success has been achieved in recent years, which almost certainly deserves a place among the most fundamental achievements of biological science.

Thus human genetics and its role in man's vulnerability to diseases may be said to have taken on a new lease on life. From perhaps a different angle it has been found that some anomalies and diseases, the causes of which were previously obscure, are now known to be connected with abnormal numbers or shapes of the chromosomes. But gene mutations do not in general show visible alterations in the chromosomes when seen under the microscope. And last but not least the study of both monozygotic and dizygotic twins has long been recognized as a fruitful field of research in human and mammalian genetics.

---

[1] Kemp (1951) describes these terms as follows: "Two essentially different factors characterizing man are heredity and environment. The hereditary factors, except in case of mutation, are transmitted unchanged from generation to generation, uninfluenced by environment. The properties characterizing individual humans depend more or less on the environment. Each of these properties manifests itself as the result of the action of one or more genes under existing conditions. The sum of these is termed the *phenotype*, or the appearance of an individual. By the *genotype*, or genetic constitution, we understand the sum of all the genes found in a single individual. The phenotype develops by the action of the environment on the genotype. The genotype is not directly visible, being in fact an abstraction."

DISEASES WITH SOME HEREDITARIAL LINKAGE

These conditions are made up of a mixed bag of defects and diseases, particularly the serious hemoglobinopathies, certain enzyme deficiencies, and inborn errors of metabolism. McKusick has designed a spectrum of some conditions, placing the diseases to which the individual is most genetically susceptible at one end, and those to which he is least susceptible at the other (see Fig. 6). Those listed at the genetic end of the scale have been estimated to affect seriously about 1 per cent of all live-born individuals at some time in their lives. The majority of these traits are dominant with a high degree of penetrance, but some are autosomal recessive and a few are sex-linked. Their clinical severity varies considerably.

It may require an unfavorable environment to bring out a given trait in a genetically susceptible population. Current investigations are revealing the changing environmental conditions under which people now live; these influence the human gene pool and, consequently, the frequencies of different genetic constitutions that determine the biological basis of the health of populations. Mental retardation is one example. A primitive pastoral community may be able to accommodate the simple-minded individual fairly well, but in an industrial community the mentally retarded may represent a burden.

There is another slant to this also, for some deleterious polymorphic traits are only prevalent in certain geographic areas or in racial groups. Thus the distribution of the sickling gene, which may give rise to sickle-cell anemia, is uneven. It is exceedingly rare in many places but the frequency of the homozygote may range between 4 and 10 per cent in some parts of Asia or Africa (*Human genetics and public health* 1964). It has been shown that the heterozygote for this trait benefits from the selective advantage of an increased resistance to malignant tertian malaria.

A list including even some of the better known examples of inherited traits thought to increase human susceptibility would be long. But I shall limit myself to the mention of one, which is

111

the slightly increased susceptibility of people possessing blood groups of the A, B, and O system to certain well-known diseases —for instance, the high probability that cancer of the stomach is about 20 per cent more frequent in persons of group A than in those belonging to group O; and the even stronger association found between group O and persons suffering from duodenal ulcer (Fraser-Roberts 1965).

RACE

The human race is of hybrid composition in general; the population of industrial cities in the United States, in particular, is polyglot in character. Criteria for determining an individual's race and nationality, not only in the United States but elsewhere, are so crude that this kind of determination is not likely to be very accurate. More usually, what is measured in this type of estimate are racial or nationality traits, whether they be due to physical attributes, customs, or local geographical conditions. Until better methods of measuring racial or ethnic types are available, it may be wiser not to attempt to separate the concept of racial susceptibility from racial habits, particularly when it comes to saying that Eskimos, American Indians, or Jews acquire this or that disease at a higher or lower rate than others.

To turn back to the epidemiologist's theoretical task of separating genotypic from phenotypic influences in a given population, I will give two examples, one in poliomyelitis and one in rheumatic heart disease. As far as I know, no special racial (genetic) susceptibility exists that would influence the rates of poliomyelitis cases to be consistently greater in one race than any other. Far more likely, if a differential rate is noted, it is due to those particular socioeconomic conditions in which that ethnic group happens to find itself.

To illustrate differing poliomyelitis rates in a population composed of different ethnic groups, one can choose for such estimates a population like that of the Hawaiian Islands, where a number of different racial stocks are represented. Since these people have more or less maintained their individual (ethnic) population groups and are listed in the Hawaiian census as such, it is easier to make differential measures of disease incidence here than elsewhere. Table 2 shows various attack rates of poliomyelitis recorded in Hawaii during the 1953–54 epidemic. That the rate for paralytic poliomyelitis in Caucasians was six times greater than in Filipinos does not mean that the ethnic (genetic) susceptibility to this disease differed by a gradient of that magnitude; the gradient probably reflects the differing customs or ways of life followed by these groups.

TABLE 2

POLIOMYELITIS ATTACK RATES IN DIFFERENT RACIAL
GROUPS IN HAWAII (1953–54) [a]

Race	Size of Population [b]	Number of Cases [c]	Rate per 100,000
Hawaiian................. (including part Hawaiian)	91,325	30	33.2
Caucasian.................	68,600	65	95.5
Chinese...................	32,052	11	34.4
Japanese..................	188,872	34	18.0
Filipino..................	62,777	10	16.1
Others [d]	21,423	6	28.5
All races............	465,325	156	29.8

[a] Data collected by Yale Poliomyelitis Study Unit from Hawaiian Territorial Department of Health before the introduction of poliomyelitis vaccine.
[b] Estimates as of July 1, 1952.
[c] Paralytic cases.
[d] "Other races" include Puerto Rican, Korean, Negro, Samoan.

Another example is that of the differences in death rates due to rheumatic heart disease between Negroes and whites in the United States (Wolff 1948). Negroes do not seem to acquire rheumatic fever at incidence rates higher than those in whites, but once acquired, this disease is more apt to be more fatal in the Negro, a feature illustrated in Fig. 19. Generally speaking, the mortality rates charted are somewhat higher among girls than boys. There is little significant difference in a statistical sense, however, except in those aged fifteen to nineteen years. In this adolescent age group, Negro females show a distinctly higher mortality than white females and Negro males. Again, this cannot except in minor degree be ascribed to racial differences, for Wolff, from whom the data in Fig. 19 were obtained, believed that Negro girls are under a greater strain at this period of life.

This was because of the greater risks of early childbearing, a situation which resembles sex differences in tuberculosis mortality in Negroes of this age. He further believed that the mortality ratios of Negro and white children, when correlated with the socioeconomic conditions under which they live, indicated that rheumatic fever and rheumatic heart disease are influenced strongly by the environment (see chap. 14). These beliefs, by the way, are based on data obtained in the years preceding 1948.

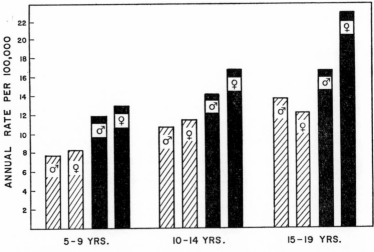

Fig. 19. Sex-specific death rates for rheumatic heart disease per 100,000 in the United States among white and Negro children and adolescents in the 1940's and before. Shaded columns represent white death rates and black columns Negro rates. In each of the three age groups shown, the mortality is higher in Negroes and, in the age group 15–19 years, this is particularly pronounced in females. (Data from Wolff, 1948. Children's Bureau Publication No. 322. Washington, D.C.)

For the present it is safer to consider that the local environment has a large share of the responsibility rather than to say that the Negro has any racial predisposition to rheumatic heart disease. The vulnerability of Negroes or Puerto Ricans who have recently moved from a rural environment to the slums of large urban cities are examples. For this reason some genetically inclined epidemiologists prefer to study remote tribes from South

America or New Guinea in their native haunts (Gajdusek 1963; Kurland 1964).

A satisfactory study of comparative racial susceptibilities to certain diseases or conditions might be made if one could divide a single ethnic group between two or three environments and compare them—Cape Verde Islanders, for instance, living on their native islands could be compared with those who have immigrated to New England cities in the United States, or Puerto Ricans with those who have immigrated to New York City. The World Health Organization Serum Bank has one or two research projects of this kind already under way.

Another example of herd susceptibility can be taken from the field of epizootiology. Twenty rams were introduced into Iceland from Europe in 1933, and soon after their introduction three destructive infectious diseases appeared in the native sheep stock, killing hundreds of thousands of the animals (Dungal *et al.* 1938, Sigurdsson 1954). None of these three diseases were known to be prevalent on the Continent, where the rams originated, but so susceptible had the sheep on Iceland become, after hundreds of years of inbreeding and freedom from exposure to foreign infectious agents, that they fell an easy prey to these "new" diseases when they were introduced by "healthy" carriers coming from a European sheep population that had been living in symbiosis with these agents. One of the agents, a virus with a long incubation period, has been identified recently and named the *Visna* virus.

SEXUAL DIFFERENCES

Many of these differences in disease acquisition and severity are too obvious to need discussion, since they are conditions based on the natural anatomical or hormonal differences between men and women. But others are more obscure. We have already mentioned that the male sex is more vulnerable to coronary occlusion than the female until after the age of 45, and that after 1920, the U.S. death rate for males failed to decline at the same rate as for females (see Fig. 15).

Some diseases are obviously the result of occupational activities. Men are more apt to be engaged in heavy work in stone quarries or mines, and as a result silicosis, anthracosis, and the various accidents prone to occur in these occupations prevail at higher rates in men than in women. There are a variety of occupational diseases in the same category, involving the so-called dangerous trades. Female occupations, too, involve distinctive risks. A young housewife with a family of several children runs a higher risk of acquiring some of the acute infectious diseases than does her husband. It is recognized, of course, that both parents have higher respiratory infection rates if and when they are exposed to young children in the home than do others, but the mother usually has the closest contact with the younger children, who may be a great source of the spread of the causative agents.

More puzzling, however, are certain other diseases, many of them of obscure etiology, that are well known to be more common in one sex for unknown reasons. The predominant prevalence of rheumatoid arthritis and lupus erythematosus disseminatus in the female are examples. No satisfactory explanation has ever been given for this differentiation, nor is it clear why men are more prone to get carcinoma of the stomach than women and why the incidence of carcinoma of the large bowel is at least as high and in many places higher among women than among men.

Family Susceptibilities

The inheritance of family traits may predispose one to such diseases as congenital anomalies, gout, hemophilia, muscular dystrophy, and bronchial asthma. Some of these afflictions are transmitted according to Mendelian principles, others do not seem to be. Here is where the application of medical or clinical genetics comes in.

One might choose the rheumatic fever family as an example where discussions have long been active as to whether genetic susceptibility existed because this disease commonly runs through more than one generation (see Fig. 25), or whether households where rheumatic fever thrives from one generation to another are hotbeds of streptococcal infection because of environmental reasons. One is constantly faced with an awareness that a high familial prevalence (aggregates of cases) in the family or domiciliary group by no means establishes a hereditary tendency to acquire this condition. Other things run in families, in which domiciliary factors or local customs determine the situation. Perhaps the most illuminating observations come from the study of identical twins who have been brought up since birth in two different environments and whose growth characteristics as well as the acquisition of illness and injuries have been carefully noted for many years.

HUMAN PHYSIQUE

This whole area of investigation requires much more measurement and study and can hardly yet be called a science. It is concerned with relationships to constitutional or physical traits and disease prevalence. Dark hair and dark skin versus blond hair and light skin is one example. Other traits include sthenic, and asthenic, and pyknic, types of human physique or, in more modern terms, the endomorph, mesomorph, and ectomorph varieties. More emphasis was placed a generation ago upon certain physical traits as characteristic measures of susceptibility (or the lack of it) to certain diseases than is done now. We would do well to examine the principles outlined by Draper (1924), Davenport (1923), and others in the 1920's on the relationships of human constitution, body build, and disease, based on anthropometric measurements on patients. Most conspicuous among these differences were those between "ectomorphic" peptic ulcer patients and "endomorphic" gall bladder patients.[2]

Finally come questions of immunity and the measurement of antibodies and skin sensitivity to a variety of agents, such as bacterial or virus antigens or allergens and their use as an index

[2] Reduced to the simplest of descriptions, taken from Sheldon's book (1940), *endomorphy* means a relative predominance of soft, rounded contours throughout various topical regions of the body. *Mesomorphy* means a relative predominance of muscle, bone, and connective tissue. *Ectomorphy* means a relative predominance of linearity and fragility.

117

of resistance or sensitivity. Far more accurate and quantitative measurements may be made here than those descriptive of body build and ways of life. The use of serological measurements in this connection has great promise. It will be taken up in the next chapter.

BIBLIOGRAPHY

DAVENPORT, C. B. 1923. *Body build, its development and inheritance.* Carnegie Institution Publication 329. Washington, D.C.

DRAPER, G. 1924. *Human constitution: A consideration of its relationship to disease.* Philadelphia: W. B. Saunders Co.

DUNGAL, N. GISLASON, G. and TAYLOR, E. L. 1938. Epizoötic adenomatosis in the lungs of sheep. *J. Comp. Path. Therap.* **51**:45–68.

FRASER-ROBERTS, J. A. 1965. ABO blood groups, secretor status, and susceptibility to chronic diseases: an example of a genetic basis for family predispositions. In *Genetics and the epidemiology of chronic diseases.* Public Health Service Publication No. 1163. Department of Health, Education, and Welfare. Washington, D.C.: Government Printing Office.

GAJDUSEK, D. C. 1963. Motor-neurone disease in natives of New Guinea. *New Engl. J. Med.* **266**:471–76.

Human genetics and public health. 1964. Technical Report 282. 2d Report of World Health Organization Expert Committee on Human Genetics. Geneva.

KEMP, T. 1951. *Genetics and disease.* London: Oliver & Boyd.

KURLAND, L. T. 1965. The geographic and genetic characteristics of amyotrophic lateral sclerosis and other selected chronic neurological diseases. In *Genetics and the epidemiology of chronic diseases.* Public Health Service Publication No. 1163. Department of Health, Education and Welfare. Washington, D.C.: Government Printing Office.

McKUSICK, V. A. 1965. Coronary artery disease. In *Genetics and the epidemiology of chronic diseases.* Public Health Service Publication No. 1163. Department of Health, Education and Welfare. Washington, D.C.: Government Printing Office.

SHELDON, W. H. 1940. *The varieties of human physique.* New York: Harper & Bros.

SIGURDSSON, B. 1954. Maedi, a slow progressive pneumonia of sheep: An epizoölogical and pathological study. *Brit. Vet. J.* **110**:225–70.

WOLFF, G. 1948. Childhood mortality from rheumatic fever and rheumatic heart disease. Publicat. 322. Washington, Department of Health, Education, and Welfare, Children's Bureau.

Serological Epidemiology

We have already mentioned in previous chapters that the immune status of the host—the condition of the "epidemiological soil, "—is of prime importance in nearly all epidemiological situations where an infectious disease is concerned. This can be tested and demonstrated experimentally in animals, particularly small animals such as mice, by actually exposing them to a dangerous agent and then watching what happens. In man, however, this demonstration has not been so easy. Nevertheless, measurements of immunity on a mass scale have become more available in the field of epidemiology. Prior to about 1900 the information about human immunity was limited to reports by individuals about whether they had been vaccinated or had had a disease, or to the presence of actual physical signs such as the scars from chicken pox. These are very limited measures, particularly because they rest upon memory or clinical evidence of past infection and do not take into account the fact that much of man's immunity is acquired subclinically through mild, unrecognized, or inapparent infection.

Around the beginning of the twentieth century, measurements about the immune status or infection status of a given population to such infectious diseases as tuberculosis and diphtheria began to be obtained from the use of skin tests like the tuberculin test and its modifications, and the Schick test. The latter was immediately used on a large scale to measure immunity against diphtheria. The use of many other tests have followed.

These skin-test surveys measure tissue reactivity, indicating the presence or absence of previous exposure and infection by a given etiologic agent. How the age-specific pattern has differed in various localities is illustrated in Fig. 20. Data by Hetherington *et al.* (1929) record results from tuberculin tests, and data by Frost (1928) from Schick tests in children of various age groups in New York City and Baltimore during the 1920's, which was a time when relatively few had been artificially immunized against diphtheria.

The use of serologic tests for disease surveys as opposed to their use to diagnose individual cases may be said to have begun with attempts to map out the distribution of syphilis in segments

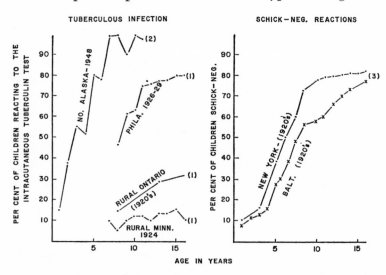

Fig. 20. Early use of tuberculin and Schick test surveys in school children, representing various localities and times. These show a wide range of results in the former. (Tuberculin test data from [1] Hetherington *et al.*, 1929. A survey to determine the prevalence of tuberculous infection in school children. *Am. Rev. Tuberc.* **20**:421; [2] personal communication from D. M. Chalmers, Alaskan Territory Department of Health, 1949; Schick test data from [3] Frost, W. H., 1928. Infection, immunity, and disease in the epidemiology of diphtheria. *J. Preventive Med.* **2**:325.)

of urban populations by means of the Wassermann test. As early as 1916, Dr. J. Whitridge Williams had begun to require a routine Wassermann test on all patients attending the prenatal clinic of the Johns Hopkins Hospital, a total averaging at that time well over a 1,000 per year (1920). It was his purpose to bring those women who needed it under treatment, as well as to increase our "knowledge concerning the incidence of the disease." It cannot be stressed too strongly that the serum survey, designed to measure the immune status of a given population reveals only those types of immunity in which antibodies develop, as opposed of course, to other types of immunity to infection in which no such development of antibodies is demonstrable.

Today the most useful human serum collections consist of random samplings obtained from normal individuals who represent defined population groups. In these samples one can measure various substances found in serum. The number and variety of such substances and the number of tests used to detect them have increased almost monthly. At present, close to 100 different determinations can be made on a single sample of whole blood, provided the volume of the specimen is adequate. Some of the measurable constituents concern the donor's genotype, such as blood groups; others represent metabolic variations or abnormalities; and still others measure immunological status, such as antibodies, which may be said to represent persistent or transient "footprints" of an infection previously experienced in the remote or recent past. The patterns revealed by the various measurements can often be correlated with broad differences in ways of living characteristic of given populations, as well as with ethnic factors.

With the serologic survey of antibodies, one must realize that, as with many skin tests, the information gained from such measurements seldom corresponds to a record of past illnesses, but rather it reflects both recognized and unrecognized infections, the great majority of which have been so mild as to put them in the second category. Thus, antibody surveys essentially can be a measure of infection rates rather than of illness rates. Only a few notable exceptions to this can be found. One is measles. Inapparent infection with measles virus seems to be rare; therefore, for that disease, illness rates, infection rates, and antibody prevalence appear to be virtually one and the same.

In the field of poliomyelitis, Aycock and Kramer (1930 *a* and *b*) were measuring antibody titers to poliovirus in attempts to map the distribution of this infection in the late 1920's; they used the cumbersome monkey intracerebral neutralization test, the only serologic method then available for studying the disease. Others pursued similar studies in the 1930's, still hampered by the lack of precise techniques. But today, as a result of methodological advances, particularly the introduction of tissue culture methods, there is hardly a civilized nation conscious of its local public health problems that has not determined the antibody patterns for each of the three types of poliovirus within segments of its juvenile population.

Figure 21 illustrates serum surveys conducted in 1949–51 and the different prevaccination patterns of Type II poliovirus antibodies in three populations. Each of these populations had been exposed to a totally different type of environment. The distribution of antibody reflects the age at which infection occurred in these populations: in early childhood in a crowded urban environment where low standards of hygiene prevailed (Cairo, Egypt); considerably later in childhood in a city with high standards of hygiene (Miami, Fla.); and not until young adult life in a small remote Arctic population (North Alaska). Differences can also be demonstrated in population groups within the same district or city by sampling different socioeconomic strata.

In the field of arboviruses, the earliest serologic surveys were conducted in the 1930's by Soper and his associates (1933) from the Rockefeller Foundation in certain South American populations. These surveys were concerned with the prevalence of antibodies to yellow fever virus. From this work came the demonstration of the existence of jungle yellow fever. By the early 1940's, the serum survey had become a well-established technique for mapping the geographic distribution of other arbovirus infections. A pioneer example was the study of mosquito-borne so-called virus encephalitis B of Japan, now familiarly known as Japanese encephalitis; it is widespread in the Far East. It was somewhat surprising to U.S. investigators to learn, very shortly after the end of World War II, that for almost a decade, Japanese virologists had been mapping the prevalence of infections with Japanese encephalitis virus in their country by mass antibody surveys using collections of sera from both man and animals (Paul and Hammon 1946). Since 1946, with the advent and increasing use of new methods, this approach has been expanded to cover a variety of old and newly discovered

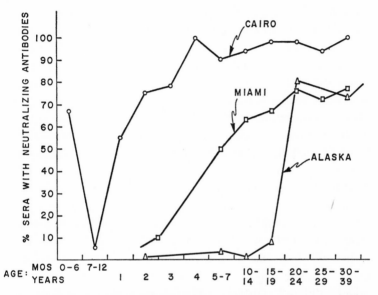

FIG. 21. Age-specific rates and patterns at which neutralizing antibodies to Type 2 poliovirus developed in three areas, 1949–51. The two cities shown—Cairo, Egypt, and Miami, Florida—are located at about the same latitude, but in 1950 they differed considerably as to sanitary arrangements as well as to the age composition of their respective populations. The Alaskan sera were from two Eskimo villages located at the extreme northwest of this state. (Cairo data from Paul, Melnick, Barnett, and Goldblum, 1952; Miami data from Paul, Melnick, and Riordan, 1952; Eskimo data from Paul and Riordan, 1950.)

arbovirus infections in widely separated parts of the world: the Soviet Union, the Philippine Islands, Malaya, Australia, India, Africa, Eastern Europe, and the entire Western Hemisphere.

The use of serum surveys as applied to infectious disease has included latterly infections caused by the viruses of measles and mumps, respiratory viruses and many other agents including parasitic agents. A major step in furthering this expansion occurred in 1961 when the World Health Organization established three Reference Serum Banks.[1] These banks have served as repositories for various collections of human sera from widely distributed sources. A major principle on which the serum banks were established was that serum collections, if properly documented and stored (generally frozen at −20° C) can serve many purposes. Some sera can be put aside for testing in future years by methods as yet undiscovered. These multiple functions for serum banks have been described in several reports, to one of which the reader is referred. This documents information to be obtained in serum surveys and discusses how results can be analyzed on age-specific, geographic, ethnic, and socioeconomic bases (Paul 1963). It may be unnecessary to point out that the degree to which serum surveys can contribute to the science of epidemiology and other ecologic sciences is yet to be fully explored.

The term serological epidemiology is not used here to describe a new or special kind of epidemiological science but to describe a method that has unique applications when it comes to comparing the health experience of various populations with widely different customs, different concepts of disease, and diagnostic criteria of illness. Serological surveys seem to be of particular value among populations that have special habits, and for which morbidity data and vital statistics are scanty or completely lacking; that is, in populations characterized by primitive health facilities and a dearth of existing medical information. Examples are the isolated, relatively inaccessible areas where collections of serum are made with difficulty, such as on the Island of Tristan da Cunha, Easter Island, or among South African bushmen, or Eskimos from North Alaska.

Importance of documentation of populations involved. Many different objectives may prompt one to make collections of sera,

[1] WHO Reference Serum Banks are at present located in Prague, Czechoslovakia, Johannesburg, South Africa, and New Haven, Connecticut.

124

but it cannot be emphasized too strongly that nearly all such collections lose much of their value if adequate descriptions of the population and records of the circumstances involved are not obtained. Not only should basic information on all individuals donating sera be recorded on a reasonably standard questionnaire but a community medical history should be taken whenever possible. This should include vital statistics and significant local demographic and epidemiologic data. Sometimes, of course, as when dealing with a primitive tribe, it is next to impossible to get anything but sketchy information. But the important point is that when the sera have eventually been tested, correct interpretations of the results may rest upon the degree of accuracy with which demographic, ecologic, and epidemiologic data have been assembled. The required basic, epidemiologic information should cover as many aspects as are feasible because of the diversity of objectives involved in the multipurpose survey and the diversity of tests that may eventually be carried out. The sampling method to be used in covering a given population is of major importance. In general, blood specimens should be collected on a random basis from normal individuals of a stated age and sex. Adequate age groups should be included (see Appendix II for example). Specimens collected from populations in hospitals and other institutions are less desirable; if for some reason it is necessary to include them, the degree of bias thus introduced should be documented. Although a true random sample is the ideal, it is seldom possible to achieve. It is essential, therefore, that the exact sampling method used in obtaining any collection be clearly defined to avoid the possibility that the collection might be used for purposes for which it is not suitable. The threat of incorrect usage of serum collections is an ever present danger.[2]

Various types of immunologic and other serum surveys. The main emphasis on the serum survey so far has been on infectious diseases. Such surveys may detect antibodies, against viral and bacterial agents and their toxins, as well as antibodies

[2] Further details about collecting sera for these purposes will be found in the Appendix II.

against protozoa and other parasites. Nevertheless the serologic approach to the study of epidemiology is by no means limited to infectious diseases and antibody patterns. This approach may have applications in a variety of fields including anthropology, genetics, and nutrition. Such surveys may deal with blood groups, the different types of hemoglobinopathies and anemias. Also, the serologic aspects of nutrition, such as the measurement of serum protein, blood vitamins and minerals, or the surveys carried out by the Interdepartmental Committee on Nutrition for National Defense (1963) are good examples. The serologic aspects of these subjects are but one part, often a minor part, of a survey. Usually they require considerably more time to be spent in the field for the examination of certain existing clinical conditions, and they often require a larger staff, including experts who are better able to cope with special fields than is the ordinary serologic epidemiologist.

Other chronic diseases. Another blood component whose prevalence has been measured in different serologic surveys is the rheumatoid factor. This is a substance of somewhat obscure significance but one known to increase with age and to be of diagnostic importance in certain active cases of rheumatoid arthritis.

Blood lipids. In considering the potentialities for illness associated with atherosclerosis, and such entities as ischemic heart disease and cerebral hemorrhages, one can trace certain relationships by means of serologic findings designed to measure lipoproteins. Major substances thought to have a quantitative relationship with ischemic heart disease and atherosclerosis include serum lipids, such as cholesterol and triglycerides. The levels of these, in turn, are influenced by race, diets, and ways of living (see chap. 19). When surveys to determine these blood lipids are contemplated in the course of a serum survey, it is well to include measurements of blood pressure and height and weight (ponderal indexes) along with the serum sampling. It is easy to see how much more time consuming and complicated this type of project can become than a simple serum survey.

Examples of Serologic Surveys. There are so many aspects of these surveys that to include them all would be quite impossible. I shall mention only three:

1. Determination of whether a given antibody or blood component can be found in a population or area, by screening representative sera for their presence. Essentially this is a preliminary, exploratory type of survey designed to lead to further work, and a true random sampling is not particularly important.
2. Determination of the prevalence of age-specific rates of antibodies or blood components in different populations or in different segments of the same population. Of course the immunization status of a population can be measured here too as in a vaccine trial, and subsequent to it. A random sample is important here.
3. Longitudinal studies, requiring serum collections to be made at sequential intervals on the same population and occasionally on matched samples during epidemics. These investigations may constitute long-term prospective studies designed to detect fluctuations in the activity of age-specific antibodies. Repeated specimens taken from members of industrial groups, or from mobile military or other units prior to departure for assignment in a foreign country and after their return, furnish examples. This is a useful method of measuring the hazards of infection in new and strange environments. Short-term studies may be focused on the immune status of the same or different members of a given population before or early in the course of an epidemic. Under such circumstances, inapparent infection and frank disease rates may be compared and examined in relation to age, various sociologic and other pertinent factors.

Limitations of Serologic Surveys. Having stated the possibilities of the serologic survey method, I must now emphasize its limitations. Most experience with this approach has been in the investigation of infectious diseases; indeed methods of applying it to most chronic diseases require much more exploration. Obviously, not all important infectious diseases lend themselves to study by means of serologic epidemiology; tuberculosis is a notable example. In other infections, antibodies may be transient; and surveys to detect them are meaningful only under those special circumstances of that particular epidemic.

Cross-reactions between antigenically related systems sometimes make the interpretation of results very difficult in the parasitic field as well as the arbovirus field. Many times the suspected specific antibody detected actually has represented a response to a closely related but different agent from the one used in the serologic test. Difficulties in technique and interpretation also arise. Needless to say, the investigator must have a thorough knowledge of the tests being used, their nonspecific reactions, limits of accuracy, and diagnostic significance. Since such large numbers of tests are required—many of them expensive—and since the volume of sera from each specimen may be limited, tests requiring small volumes of blood are at a premium. If quantitative determinations are to be made, often arbitrary decisions are required to define what is to be called a positive test, and what are the limits of normal values. Obviously the reproducibility and sensitivity of the tests in the hands of different investigators is also a crucial point.

Furthermore, although an earlier section of this chapter has been devoted to problems of sampling large and small communities, the necessity of avoiding bias in the selection of any population must be re-emphasized, particularly if antibody rates are to be estimated.

In summary, it should be stressed that this method of serologic survey holds out great promise for accurate assay of immunological status and comparative measures between populations that may have widely different cultural patterns. Nevertheless, even though some of the uses of serum surveys have been adequately demonstrated, the method is still being explored. The next decade should testify far more to the value of such surveys in dealing with epidemiological problems than any estimate that can be given now.

BIBLIOGRAPHY

AYCOCK, W. L. and KRAMER, S. D. 1930*a*. Immunity to poliomyelitis in normal individuals in urban and rural communities as indicated by the neutralization test. *J. Prev. Med.* 4:189–200.

———. 1930*b*. Immunity to poliomyelitis in a southern population as shown by the neutralization test. *Ibid.* 201–6.

FROST, W. H. 1928. Infection, immunity, and disease in the epidemiology of diphtheria. *J. Prev. Med.* 2:325–43.

HETHERINGTON, H. W., MCPHEDRAN, F. M., LANDIS, H. R. M., and

OPIE, E. L. 1929. A survey to determine the prevalence of tuberculous infection in school children. *Am. Rev. Tuber.* **20**:421–510.

Interdepartmental Committee on Nutrition for National Defense. 1963. Manual for nutrition surveys. 2d ed. Washington, D.C.: Government Printing Office.

PAUL, J. R. 1963. The aims and purposes of World Health Organization serum banks. *Yale J. Biol. Med.* **36**:2–5.

PAUL, J. R. and HAMMON, W. M. 1946. Report submitted to the Army Epidemiological Board and to the Surgeon General of the U.S. Army (Washington). Unpublished.

PAUL, J. R., MELNICK, J. L., BARNETT, V., and GOLDBLUM, N. A. 1952. Survey of neutralization antibodies to poliomyelitis virus in Cairo, Egypt. *Amer. J. Hyg.* **55**:402–13.

PAUL, J. R., MELNICK, J. L. and RIORDAN, J. T. 1952. Comparative neutralizing antibody patterns to Lansing (Type 2) poliomyelitis virus in different populations. *Amer. J. Hyg.* **56**:232–51.

PAUL, J. R. and RIORDAN, J. T. 1950. Observations on serological epidemiology: Antibodies to the Lansing strain of poliomyelitis virus in sera from Alaskan Eskimos. *Amer. J. Hyg.* **52**:202–12.

SOPER, F. L., PENNA, H., CARDOSO, E., SERAFIN, J., FROBISHER, M., and PINHEIRO, J. 1933. Yellow fever without *Aëdes aeygpti:* Study of a rural epidemic in the Valle do Chanaan, Espirito Santo, Brazil, 1932. *Amer. J. Hyg.* **18**:555–87.

WILLIAMS, J. W. 1920. The value of the Wassermann reaction in obstetrics, based upon the study of 454 consecutive cases. *Johns Hopkins Hosp. Bull.* **31**:335–42.

CHAPTER XIII

The Environment: Geographic Pathology

In this chapter we are concerned with the geographical distribution of various diseases as well as with their behavior in different places. This may deal with the effects of living in crowded cities as opposed to remote islands or with diseases of tropical jungles or arid wastes. But, in general, geographical medicine or pathology deals directly or indirectly with the effects of climate and location on epidemiology and other aspects of human disease and human behaviour, a subject treated so well by Dubos (1965), in his book *Man Adapting*.

Epidemiologic climates may be of two types: microclimates, described as sociologic climates, representing intimate living conditions within the home or place of work; and macroclimates, which represent climate in the ordinary, meteorologic sense:— temperature, moisture, and rainfall. It is with the more familiar macroclimate that we will first be concerned.

HISTORICAL NOTE

The idea that certain places are endowed with salubrious climates and others are not can be traced at least as far back as Hippocrates' treatise *On Airs, Waters and Places* (1886 translations by Francis Adams). It has concerned physicians ever since, and by the eighteenth century, medical climatology had already become a subject for textbooks.

Geographic pathology, considered in an epidemiologic sense as opposed to a therapeutic sense, started with the work of August Hirsch in 1860. In its subsequent development (Davidson, 1892, and Clemow, 1903), work in the field of tropical medicine perhaps had the largest share. But a major contributing influence was the writings of Ellsworth Huntington (1915) and Bryan (1933). Although they did not contribute to the medical story particularly, they were responsible for generating a great deal of general interest. The medical aspect was broadened when many authors had the perspicacity to concern themselves not merely with the geography and climatology of diseases and their prevalence in different places, but with the shifting character of disease in various places, which changed as the customs and habits of the various inhabitants changed (Dieuaide, 1945). Actually the idea of geomedicine as an epidemiologic discipline still lagged for half a century or more. Within the past generation,[1] however, it has again come into its own, partly because of the work of the World Health Organization. Many others have been interested recently including Jacques May (1950, 1961) and Dudley Stamp whose *Geography of Health and Disease* has been put out in paperback (1964).

PRESENT CONCEPTS OF GEOGRAPHIC PATHOLOGY

This coming of age of geomedicine has been due not only to the development of new concepts of the pathogenesis of disease and to new methods for measuring the prevalence of disease, but also to the fact that the world has grown smaller and that there are more international organizations vitally concerned today with health and preventive medicine than before. Furthermore, industrial and other interests have been anxious to solve new problems of health and productivity in the tropics or other

[1] During World War II considerable attention was given to geographical medicine. An *Atlas of Disease* known as the *Welt-Seuchen-Atlas*, was prepared in Germany under military auspices. This has subsequently been published in a second and more extended edition under the title *World Atlas of Epidemic Diseases* (1951–56). In the United States a series of volumes on *Global Epidemiology* have appeared since 1946 (Simmons *et al.*) as the result of efforts of the Preventive Medicine Service in the Office of the Surgeon General of the U.S. Army. The American Geographical Society has also taken a leading part (Light 1944) in this movement by the publication of a series of maps, edited by May (1950, 1961) illustrating the distribution of various diseases.

remote areas heretofore neglected. This calls for a reappraisal of health conditions by up-to-date methods. It takes little imagination to visualize what forms this appraisal might take in reviewing features that the tropical epidemiologist would wish to measure, those ecologic conditions that promote the spread of malaria, yellow fever, intestinal infections, hepatitis, food spoilage, and parasitic infestations. The effects of extreme cold and prolonged heat, particularly moist heat, on the human body, and associated salt depletion of the body are also manifestations of how man's health may be directly affected by climates. Such effects may also be indirect, reflecting ways of living and habits gradually adopted by populations brought up under conditions ranging from arctic to tropical.

The general scope of geographical medicine calls for more than listing data on the presence or prevalence of special or exotic diseases in various parts of the world. It calls for a study of the local peculiarities of diseases and the factors that aid or interfere with recovery from illness. These may differ greatly from place to place. Geomedicine also includes comparisons of the clinical picture of a given disease as it occurs in various places. This may mean a comparison of a disease in natives as opposed to the same disease which one might see in visitors to the area.

For instance, natives living in a very remote part of the world may be less resistant to tuberculosis than other populations. Under such circumstances, the childhood type of tuberculosis may develop in native adults, previously unexposed to tubercle bacilli, and result in a kind of tuberculosis far more devastating than the usual adult type. The effect "civilization" has had in bringing about the astronomically high infantile rate of positive tuberculin tests in Eskimos bears witness to this (see Fig. 20). The serious impact of influenza epidemics upon Eskimo populations is another example; apparently the same type and strain of influenza virus can cause a mild illness in southern Canada and a disease with high mortality among Eskimo populations in the Far North. Furthermore, the high rate of paralytic disease in poliomyelitis epidemics among adult Eskimos is proverbial. These are but a few of the many examples which illustrate geographical characteristics of an infectious disease in remote places.

CLIMATE AND ITS DIRECT EFFECTS

If we arbitrarily assume that temperate climates represent the norm, then extremes or even moderate deviations of warmth or cold, of aridity or humidity can greatly effect man's physiologic activities and his health. Climate influences the capacity or the inclination of man for physical activity under various temperatures, salt depletion in hot climates, and a desire for high caloric (high fat) diets in some of the colder lands. So numerous are various examples that it hardly warrants going into them here. And yet to indicate how obscure the nature of this relationship with climate may be one might cite the degree to which the incidence of multiple sclerosis (a disease of unknown cause) seems to be more common in northern than in southern latitudes. It is a striking example of the effect of climate having to do with a common disorder of mysterious nature, whose etiology conceivably might be solved by taking advantage of this fact.

ALTITUDE

Living conditions in mountainous areas or on high plateaus also have epidemiologic aspects. Reduced oxygen tension in the atmosphere, which can produce acute distress in those not acclimated to this condition, is but one example. New discoveries, which have been coming on apace as a result of high-altitude laboratories and space-age studies, are bringing us up to date on this, although we still have much to learn.

In a different vein the relationship between high altitude and the prevalence of streptococcal infections has come to the fore. This was brought home forcibly to the American armed forces during World War II, when it became apparent that the populations in large military camps in Colorado and Idaho sustained higher rates for streptococcal infections than elsewhere. The nature of this relationship is not known, but it is suspected that atmospheric and climatic conditions at these altitudes are either peculiarly conducive to the dissemination of streptococci from one individual to another or that these conditions render the tissues of the host more susceptible. This increase in streptococcal infections at high altitudes automatically increases the prevalence of the late effects of these infections in the form of rheumatic fever, as high mortality rates from rheumatic fever occur in the mountain states of the United States and Mexico City (see chap. 15).

SOIL CONDITIONS

Iodine deficiency in the soil in certain areas has an effect upon the morphology of the thyroid gland. Goiters associated with iodine deficiency are frequent among mountain dwellers in the

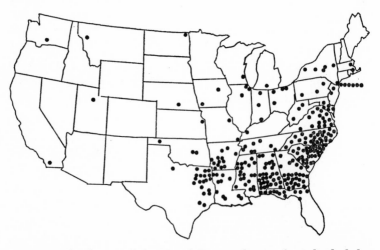

FIG. 22. Sketch map of the United States indicating by individual dots the birthplaces of 270 servicemen who contracted sarcoidosis in World War II. (Redrawn from data recorded by Gentry *et al.*, 1955. Studies on the epidemiology of sarcoidosis in the United States: the relationship to soil areas and to urban-rural residence. *J. Clin. Invest.* **34:**1839.)

Alps and the Andes, and, in some areas, are almost universal among the older age groups. There are other characteristics of soils, or more appropriately of the "mineral environment"; for instance, certain tribes in central Africa have a craving for salt, whereas Eskimos show a decided distaste for it.

Since 1932 it has been appreciated that a high fluorine content in the soil of certain localities was related to a condition of the teeth known as mottled enamel. The role that the lack of fluorine plays in the prevalence of dental caries was demonstrated in 1937 (Van Burkalow 1946).

In the realm of infectious disease a case in point would be the association with the dry and dusty plains of Arizona and parts of California, which make soil conditions particularly favorable for the dissemination of coccidiomycosis infections. Indeed, the relationship of mycotic infections to vegetation and growing conditions would yield numerous examples.

An obscure relationship occurs as regards the geographical distribution of sarcoidosis (Boeck's sarcoid) in the United States. The study by Gentry *et al.* (1955) and earlier observations by Michael *et al.* (1950) have demonstrated a concentration of cases in the southeastern part of the United States (see Fig. 22). Gentry employed random sampling in determining the birth-place of 290 patients with sarcoidosis, which had been recognized in United States servicemen during World War II. The etiology and pathogenesis of this chronic disease is unknown, and, correspondingly, the explanation of this extraordinary geographical distribution is also unknown. It has been conjectured that the soil types in the regions of high prevalence are in part responsible and that residence in rural areas of the southeast, particularly regions with fine sandy soil, offer local ecological conditions apparently favorable to the development of this peculiar disease. Obviously, for a proper evaluation of the implications of the spot map one should have some knowledge of the denominators, in this situation namely, the population distribution in the United States as well as the distribution of Negroes. For one could ask with good reason whether the map reflects racial concentration of this disease in the Negro population of the United States, considering that sarcoidosis is much more common in Negroes. According to Gentry, however, the concentration of dots in Fig. 22 does reflect a true higher prevalence in the southeast, and the racial factor is only a partial explanation for this geographical distribution.

Recently, another explanation was proposed by Cummings and Hudgins (1958). They suggest that the pollen of pine trees, which are prevalent in the endemic area, is sufficiently similar to some of the chemical constituents of the tubercle bacilli to cause the granulomatous lesions of Boeck's sarcoid in those who are adequately exposed.

ISOLATED AREAS

Still another and a most important consideration in the field of geomedicine is the geographically isolated population. An example is Arctic medicine, a new field for the epidemiologist. Isolated populations, particularly Arctic populations, today often suffer from a limited food supply. They seem to suffer less from hunger and cold, however, than they do from the sudden encroachment of civilization, which brings, among other things, breakfast food and candy, firearms and alcohol, spirochaetes, bacteria, and viruses, with which many Eskimos have had little or no previous contact. The epidemiology of disease and injury caused by these innovations is not so different from that of any population which has escaped exposure for years. The devastating epidemics of poliomyelitis and influenza among Eskimos in the Canadian Arctic (Peart 1949) bear witness to this. Another instance was Joseph Aronson's [*] observations on the prevalence of tuberculous infection among Alaskan Eskimos, which in one village in the 1930's and 1940's a rate of positive tuberculin tests reaching 95 per cent in infants under five years of age was found (see Fig. 20).

The size of the isolated population is a most important factor in considerations of the maintenance or endemicity of a given acute infection or infectious agent for which there is no extrahuman host. Such is the case with measles virus. If the population is small, geographically remote, and particularly if it consists of separated groups living in scattered villages, an acute infection will soon burn itself out, and the infectious agent may disappear completely and remain absent, perhaps for years, until reintro-

[*] J. Aronson 1949: personal communication.

duced by some outsider. This gives little or no opportunity for latent immunization to develop in the interim. Actually this was the situation along the eastern seaboard of colonial America in the seventeenth century, when measles epidemics were widely separated in point of time but devastating when precipitated by the arrival of infected people. The same situation has occurred recently in the isolated villages along the Labrador Coast, and it is familiar in the South Sea Islands.

The inability of a common infection to maintain itself in an isolated population of relatively small size was well documented on the island of Spitzbergen some twenty-five years ago by Paul and Freese (1933). At a time when the only means of communication with the outside world was by boat, a long winter from October until May completely isolated the island because of ice conditions. During these periods "colds," or at least certain acute upper respiratory infections, disappeared from the island whose population, numbering several hundred, was apparently not large enough to support the causative respiratory viruses as a source of endemic infection. Perhaps it was a matter of chance that there happened to be no chronic carriers of the viruses on the island. In any event, with the arrival of the first boat each spring, the annual epidemic of colds would sweep the island.

TROPICAL DISEASE

It is obvious that the field of tropical disease is geographical medicine in the sense that its quota of viral, bacterial and parasitic infestations owe their existence to the degree with which the etiologic agent depends for its ecology on tropical conditions. A parasite illustrative of these conditions is that which gives rise to a very common condition known as—schistosomiasis. It is responsible for illness in vast areas of the world—Africa, the Caribbean area, and northern South America to mention but a few. In many of these areas the irrigation ditches are the breeding places for the snails that maintain one of the larval stages of the parasite. When children play or adults work in these ditches with bare feet and legs they are readily infested.

137

This parasite causes a disease that is often serious and in certain forms gives rise to lesions associated with cancer.

ROLE OF INSECT VECTORS AND THEIR ECOLOGY

Geographical medicine deals with more than physical geography and the local inhabitants and their habits. The entire flora and fauna of a place may be involved, and this can be a very complicated cosmos indeed. Where certain insect vectors thrive and carry the appropriate parasites, whether they be protozoa, bacteria, or viruses, and where the appropriate mammalian or avian hosts exist, there certain insect-borne diseases are found. Among these are infections caused by arthropod-borne viruses of yellow fever, dengue, and encephalitis; and other agents, such as malaria, plague, and the rickettsioses. Conditions for the spread of some insect-borne diseases are limited to a relatively small territory, such as the concentration of veruga peruana on the west side of the Andes. This limitation is usually considered to be due to the range of the insect vector which calls for very special ecologic conditions. With malaria, enormous areas are covered or at least were covered prior to the onset of the intensive mosquito abatement programs which have reduced the prevalence of malaria since World War II.

The distribution of yellow fever, a mosquito-borne disease, introduces some extraordinary problems in geographic epidemiology. May (1961) has mapped the presence of this serious disease, along with dengue fever, in Africa and South and Central America and to a lesser extent in other parts of the world; he utilized in large measure data collected by the World Health Organization. This mapping has not only recorded the presence and location of human cases but, in the case of yellow fever, has been aided by a search for the presence of specific antibodies in the serum of man and animals.

Yellow fever and dengue fever are viral infections caused by a subgroup of a family of viruses that bear certain immunologic relationships to one another. Both can be transmitted to man through the agency of the same mosquito, although the spectrum of natural mosquito vectors for yellow fever is broader than that for dengue. The best-known vector that transmits both yellow fever and dengue is the *Aedes aegypti* mosquito, and one might speculate that where this mosquito flourishes one will find yellow fever and dengue to an equal degree. This turns out to be only partially true. The epidemiologic situation probably involves far more than the mere presence of the insect vector or vectors. With dengue, the cycle of transmission is man-to-mosquito-to-man, even though monkeys are known to be infected in nature. With yellow fever, transmission can occur in the same way, but there is another cycle in which non-human mammalian hosts, notably monkeys, serve as a reservoir of virus. Two epidemic patterns result from this: urban yellow fever, often a "man-to-man" affair, and sylvatic (jungle) yellow fever in which non-human hosts govern distribution. The geography of these two epidemiologically related viral diseases shows special and unique features. Yellow fever in the Eastern hemisphere is limited almost entirely to a broad belt in Africa, extending right across the middle of that continent and covering some 25 degrees of latitude. Dengue is also common in this belt in Africa but not nearly as common as in other areas in Asia or the East Indies. Apparently the conditions are peculiarly adequate for the survival of yellow fever virus in this African area. It can be compared with another vast area in Brazil and the northern countries of South America, where jungle yellow fever also flourishes along with dengue. In great contrast, however, is the complete absence of yellow fever in Asia, the East Indies, Australia, and some of the Pacific Islands. Dengue is common there, and certainly the yellow fever virus vector, *A. aegypti,* is there and active in its transmission of dengue. There are several possible explanations for this, all of which involve questions of cross-immunity between these two related viral infections in man or in monkeys or even in the mosquito, but these are still theoretical.

How this information can be brought to bear on the question of control is not certain, for, although yellow fever is not the menace it used to be, the dream that it might be eliminated from the face of the earth has not yet come true. The story that presents a number of complex epidemiologic problems is still unfinished.

BIBLIOGRAPHY

ACHESON, E. D. 1961. Multiple sclerosis in British Commonwealth countries in the southern hemisphere. *Brit. J. Prevent. and Social Med.* 15:118–25.

ADAMS, FRANCIS (trans.) 1886. *The genuine works of Hippocrates.* I. New York: Wm. Wood & Co.

BRYAN, P. W. 1933. *Man's adaptation of nature.* New York: Henry Holt & Co.

CLEMOW, F. G. 1903. *The geography of disease.* London: Cambridge University Press.

CUMMINGS, M. M. and HUDGINS, P. C. 1958. Chemical constituents of pine pollen and their possible relationship to sarcoidosis. Abstract in *J. Clin. Invest.* 37:888.

DAVIDSON, A. 1892. *Geographical pathology.* Edinburgh: Young J. Pentland.

DIEUAIDE, F. R. 1945. Tropical disease and geopathology. *Science* 102:656.

DUBOS, R. 1965. *Man adapting.* New Haven: Yale University Press.

GENTRY, J. T. NITOWSKY, H. M. and MICHAEL, M. 1955. Studies on the epidemiology of sarcoidosis in the United States: The relationship to soil areas and to urban-rural residence. *J. Clin. Invest.* 34: 1839.

HIRSCH, A. 1860. *Handbuch der historisch-geographischen Pathologie.* Erlangen: Ferdinand Enke.

HUNTINGTON, E. 1915. *Civilization and climate.* New Haven: Yale University Press.

LIGHT, R. U. 1944. The progress of medical geography. Includes bibliography of medical geography covering the years 1790–1935. *Geograph. Rev.* 34:636.

MAY, J. M. 1950. Medical geography: Its methods and objectives. *Geograph. Rev.* 40:9.

———. 1961. *Studies in disease ecology.* New York: Hafner Publishing Co.

MICHAEL, M., COLE, R. M., BEESON, P. B., and OLSEN, B. J. 1950. Sarcoidosis: Preliminary report of 350 cases with special reference to epidemiology. *Am. Rev. Tuber. Pulmonary Diseases* 62:403.

PAUL, J. H. and FREESE, H. L. 1933. Epidemiological and bacteriological study of "common cold" in isolated Arctic community (Spitzbergen). *Am. J. Hyg.* 17:517.

PEART, A. F. W. 1949. An outbreak of poliomyelitis in Canadian Eskimos in wintertime; epidemiological features. *Can. J. Public Health* 40:405–17.

RODENWALDT, E. 1952–56. *World atlas of epidemic diseases.* Parts I, II, and III. Hamburg: Falk-Verlag.

SIMMONS, J. S., WHAYNE, T. F., ANDERSON, G. W., and HORACK, H. M. 1944, 1950, 1955. *Global epidemiology: A geography of disease and sanitation.* Vols. I–III. Philadelphia: J. B. Lippincott Co.

STAMP, L. D. 1964. *The geography of life and death.* Ithaca: Cornell University Press.

VAN BURKALOW, A. 1946. Fluorine in the United States water supplies. *Geograph. Rev.* 36:177.

CHAPTER XIV

The Environment: Microclimate

Microclimates have already been mentioned and briefly defined. These are the social climates of various peoples and lands, their ways of life or habits, and the local environment of homes or workshops. Such climates can differ enormously within a small area that harbors rich and poor, luxurious and squalid living. Their impacts upon disease and mortality is what Ryle has called "social pathology" (1948), and it is with this intimate, sociologic or occupational approach to epidemiology that we will deal in this chapter. Some of the obvious historical examples from the nineteenth century and before are louse-borne typhus among prison populations and scurvy among sailors during long sea voyages. Others are rheumatic fever, as it existed in the London slums during the 1920's, and pellagra in our own rural south. From the occupational standpoint, disease patterns are understandably different among factory workers and stonecutters than ministers and gardeners.

HISTORY

This discipline of social pathology seems to be almost as old as that of geographical epidemiology. Certainly the Bible and the works of Hippocrates and Galen refer to ways of preserving one's health by observing rules of health and by watching one's habits. By the eighteenth century Cheyne's *Essay on Health* (1725), which consisted of admonitions, particularly concerning food and drink, exercise and rest, the value of acquiring a hobby, and rules for the studious, was so widely read in England that it ran into many editions. But the impression one gets is that Cheyne benefited only those who were rich or intelligent enough to buy his book and to carry out his instructions. His place in medical history, most critics agree is a minor one. He wrote advice on healthful living at a time when such admonition was urgently needed (Viets 1949), but hardly less than it is today. In keeping with British eighteenth-century tradition, it was written essentially for the upper classes. Medicine as a social discipline was a long time coming of age. The bad effects that life in the slums had on human health had existed for centuries before disease was related to poor living conditions or before public attempts were made to rectify conditions.

The idea that these principles might apply to the masses or be readily available to all did not come into its own in England until the nineteenth century, when William Farr began to study the differential mortality rates in various parts of England. "He never wearied," according to Greenwood (1948), "in stressing the correlation between rates of mortality and density of population, and he shares with John Snow the honour of demonstrating statistically the correlation between mortality from cholera and pollution of water supplies." The mid-nineteenth century was, therefore, a turning point. There was a great need for social reform that was obvious at first only to a few indefatigable leaders, such as Chadwick and Simon. They fought against odds for better water supplies, slum clearance, better housing, better labor conditions in an age which regarded these efforts as local benevolences more than as efforts to develop social machinery that would insure to every individual in the community a standard of living adequate for the maintenance of health. Before this period of social awakening, public opinion might have condoned G. B. Shaw's epigram—"the trouble with the poor is poverty."

That it should have required a statistician to lead these reforms may seem strange, but facts turned out to be more convincing than words. As sanitary measures were introduced into certain districts in the 1850's, Farr pointed out that year by year a fall in mortality went along with these improvements, demonstrating the useful effects of such reforms. In any event, the growth and appreciation of "social pathology" was stimulated by the advent of statistical methods, and workers in this field have leaned heavily upon them ever since (Greenwood 1948).

The late John Ryle, a distinguished British clinician and Director of the Institute of Social Medicine at Oxford University, deserves a place in history. He was an exponent of this subject in the latter years of his life (Ryle 1948), and he used the term social pathology to describe a discipline that attempted in both an academic and a clinical sense to relate disease prevalence to social conditions. His approach was that of the clinical epidemiologist and the clinical investigator using epidemiological methods. Ryle was interested in how a variety of influences was instrumental in bringing about acute and chronic illness and in interfering with the recovery from illness. His approach represented an endeavor concerned first with the diagnosis of disease, and next with measurements of its frequency and trends within a given population or component groups of that population. This principle he regarded as demanding clinical as well as sociological and statistical judgment. His significant contribution to medicine was that he did not regard this work as an exotic specialty, or as an endeavor in the field of hygiene, or social reform in a welfare state, but as part of the doctor's job. He set forth his views on social pathology in the language of the clinician and medical professor that he was—a clinician apparently about to perform a physical examination upon a community. This brought the subject back from the administrative spheres of social reform into the laps of practicing physicians. He and others who came after him urged its recognition and study by university departments of both clinical and social medicine, pointing out that this, the technique of clinical epidemiology, is one to which physicians, as well as health officers, cannot long remain indifferent.

Today social reform has become the keynote of the age. Contrasts between rich and poor in living conditions, habits, and diets are much less in some countries at least, than they were even half a century ago. Nevertheless we are in danger that in spite of great strides made in the way of slum clearance, redevelopment and anti-poverty campaigns we may be only beginning to apprehend fundamental factors contributing to poverty and deprivations.

MAN-MADE ENVIRONMENTS

In studying the microclimate, the epidemiologist becomes concerned with measurements of the frequency, or absence, or severity of diseases in a community or within component groups of such a community. Correlations of this frequency with special features of the environment, such as local housing, occupations, and other social conditions are usually related to income levels. In some communities of appropriate size, the population can be divided into socioeconomic groups or occupational groups, each with ways of living sufficiently distinct to provide data on differential death rates or sickness rates due to tuberculosis or rheumatic fever, gastric ulcer or coronary artery disease among different strata of society.

Such analyses have indicated that disease potentialities are associated not only with age but with ways of living, working, and eating habits. Many of these factors are characteristic of both the host and the environment; many can only be described in such simple terms as the relation between water supply and bowel infections, living space and respiratory infections, income level and nutrition and growth. Many are obscure.

As an example one may compare ways of life in the United States to those in other parts of the world. The differences were manifest during World War II when American troops were suddenly introduced, not only to wartime conditions in North Africa and the Philippines, but to ordinary urban life in those areas. Here macroclimatic changes played their part, but as recent immigrants to lands that had sub-standard sanitary requirements, the soldiers had to contend with living conditions that were, to say the least, not what they had been used to. In spite of many immunization procedures and apart from the threat of exotic diseases such as malaria, dengue, and sand-fly fever, these soldiers were a prime group of "susceptible immigrants," vulnerable to acute hepatitis, poliomyelitis, and a host of diarrheal diseases. With local acclimatization, "seasoning," this picture changed, but not until the troops had acquired the above-mentioned infections at far higher rates than they would have in normal circumstances (Paul 1949).

MORTALITY AND MORBITY IN RELATION TO SOCIAL CLASS

The gradients in social classes have been emphasized in previous chapters and will be again in connection with differen-

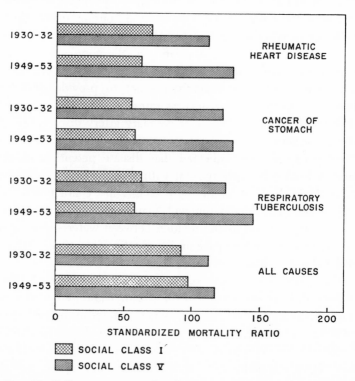

FIG. 23. Differences in mortality between men, aged 20–64 years, of different social classes in England and Wales. The experience of all these men in all classes together in each period = 100; a ratio, standardized for differences in age composition, is calculated for each social class. (Data from Morris, J. N, 1964. *Uses of epidemiology,* 2d ed., p. 58. Edinburgh: E. & S. Livingstone.)

tial rates of illness and mortality. The British are in a better position than we are to study this situation, and so I have chosen two examples from that country. There is no dearth of social inequality in the United States, but the information about it happens to be more difficult to obtain.

Morris (1964) has recorded differential mortality rates based on social classes that existed in the periods of 1930–32 and 1949–53 for certain diseases in England (see Fig. 23). Five classes of population have been recognized by the British census; No. I is the best social class, and No. V is the worst. Whatever the reasons may be, it seems clear that within the framework of this observation Class I in Britain lived longer than Class V.

RHEUMATIC FEVER AND LIVING CONDITIONS

Another British study is given as an example of the relationship of social and economic conditions to the incidence of a specific disease, rheumatic heart disease. The University of Bristol, England, in 1937 investigated the circumstances of a random sample (one family in twenty-two) of the Bristol working-class population. From the available data, the incidence of rheumatic heart disease was compared with income and with crowding in the home. These are but two aspects related to microclimate that might have been chosen, but these conditions are sometimes easier to measure than are certain other aspects, such as housing construction, dampness, and nutrition.

A total of 341 rheumatic families were selected for this study (Daniel 1942). These were divided into eight classes on the basis of net income and the number of rooms per person within the home. The number of rheumatic families in each class was divided by the number of families from a sample of the total working-class population in the same class, and to facilitate comparison of incidence between the classes, the result was expressed as a percentage of the proportion between all 341 rheumatic families and 1,424 families in the total population sample. This gave for each class the incidence of the disease as a percentage of the average income level as well as the crowding indexes among the entire population studied. The data are shown in Table 3.

The significance of the study rested largely upon the adequacy of the diagnostic criteria, the use of proper random sampling techniques, and careful statistical analyses. From these data it was concluded that: differences in incidence of rheumatic heart disease between sections of this population were associated with (1) differences in the family income; and (2) considerable differences in incidence corresponded closely with the variation in the number of rooms used by each family divided by the number of persons in the family. It was further concluded that each of these relations was true independently of the others.

TABLE 3

(1) INCIDENCE OF RHEUMATIC HEART DISEASE
IN RELATION TO NET INCOME

Net Income (as a percentage of minimum needs)	Families with Rheumatic Heart Disease	Families in Sample of Total Working-class Population	Incidence of Rheumatic Disease (as a percentage of average incidence)
Under 100	77	232	139
100–120	54	152	148
120–40	51	191	112
140–60	33	192	72
160–80	37	192	81
180–200	31	149	87
200–220	17	93	76
220 and over	41	223	77
Total	341	1,424	...

(2) INCIDENCE OF RHEUMATIC HEART DISEASE IN
RELATION TO NUMBER OF ROOMS PER PERSON

Rooms per Person	Families with Rheumatic Heart Disease	Families in Sample of Total Working-class Population	Incidence of Rheumatic Disease (as a percentage of average incidence)
Under 0.6	52	130	167
0.6–0.8	69	193	149
0.8–1.0	53	194	114
1.0–1.2	73	335	91
1.2–1.4	59	303	81
1.4–1.6	10	71	59
1.6–1.8	19	138	58
1.8 and over	6	60	42
Total	341	1,424	...

Data and terminology from Daniel, 1942.

In general this would confirm the old contention, previously based on less definite grounds, that rheumatic fever actually deserves to be called a "social disease," and it belongs in the broad category of diseases that flourish best under poor urban living conditions. Of these social aspects we will hear more later in the next chapter, which deals with rheumatic fever.

Further Examples of the Effect of Microclimate

Housing and slum clearance reforms that have concerned city health and welfare officers in the past two decades certainly represent efforts to improve local microclimates. How effective such efforts have been, aided by others that have attempted to alleviate poverty, remains to be seen. They may not have been of major concern or have seriously touched the lives of most physicians. But obviously the medical profession has been aware of the extent of such activities in urban renewal that have been going on recently and in which medical advice will be increasingly needed.

Not only have urban communities been active in providing new housing, but there has been much concern about the growing problems of pollution as well. Public health officials have been repeatedly reminding urban communities that they have "fouled their own nest," by encouraging uncontrolled industrial development. They are referring generally to water pollution, which in the United States has become shameful.

But industrial communities face another problem—that of air pollution. There are certain local geographical conditions, many of which are associated with low altitudes, that are known to promote smog. But topography is not all to blame, for a great responsibility has to be borne by the industrial plants themselves within a municipal area. The better-known air-polluted areas are London, Donora, Pennsylvania, and the Meuse Valley in Belgium. But many industrial cities have suffered from smog or are rapidly becoming victims of it. It is said that today on every square mile of New York's metropolitan area an average of 60 tons of heavy dust falls per month. The commonest offenders are fumes due to a combination of sulfur dioxide, particles of iron oxide, silicates and carbon, all common to factory smoke. Another hazard is the automobile exhaust in the city's streets.

London has been historically associated with fog—and later with smog. In December, 1952, a smog disaster claimed 4,000 lives. Ten years later a similar but less severe incident was responsible for the death of 340 Londoners. These excess deaths were, as in the earlier smog episode, all ascribed to influenza-pneumonia and cardiac illness for want of more accurate etiologic diagnoses.

INDUSTRIAL OR OCCUPATIONAL MEDICINE

Another field is prominent in any industrial civilization and offers the challenge, or the opportunity, of examining the natural history of disease in an industrial population, factory, or mine, where the workers need protection and where new hazards are constantly being uncovered, not the least of which is radiation. This activity ordinarily comes under the heading of industrial hygiene, which is so well set forth in Alice Hamilton's book *Exploring the Dangerous Trades* (1943). This field has attracted the interest of epidemiologists too (Gafafer 1943, Reid 1954). This study of factory epidemiology can be pursued when a large industrial plant is under some type of medical supervision. For one thing the population of the plant is known, and it is often easier to classify people according to the character of their jobs than to give them a purely socioeconomic rating.

An obvious correlation in this field would be the relationship between types of work and illness due to industrial diseases per se. The characteristic dermatitis that afflicts those working with cutting oils or industrial chemicals, radium poisoning, benzol poisoning, intoxications from exposure to chlorinated hydrocarbon compounds often found in solvents, and a long list of other concerns of industrial medicine represent a branch of toxicology that has become a specialty in its own right. But although the protection of the worker comes first, this discipline should not deal only with its immediate therapeutic aspects. It should deal with the more subtle aspects of industrial medicine—the character, degree, and rates of common illnesses that people in different occupations acquire, such as heart disease, respiratory infections, and gastric ulcer (Doll and Avery-Jones 1952). What may be needed in this type of epidemiological enquiry is a working population large enough to produce cases of the disease or diseases under study within a reasonable time and stable enough to maintain itself over the intended period of time. Furthermore, only comprehensive studies of industrial communities, including past and present workers, the employed and unemployed, the fit and disabled, have made it possible to reach certain conclusions or estimates of the degree of damage which the actual work inflicts upon the industrial population.

Although this is a most productive field of epidemiological research, it is also full of pitfalls. An example, which might be mentioned, is the investigation by Stewart and Hughes (1949, 1951) of tuberculosis in the boot and shoe industry. They concluded that tuberculosis was more common in this kind of industry, because, since the work was suitable for them, more people with arrested tuberculosis were engaged in this occupation; it would stand to reason then that the rate of recurrence would be higher than in the general population.

Another example of ready misinterpretation occurred in an analysis of factors other than disease severity that can contribute to absence from work. In a New England industry, whose employees are under careful medical supervision, production work is generally laborious, with lifting and carrying weights up to two hundred pounds and pushing and pulling burdens of several tons. The total absentee rate for all causes among production workers, however, was only about 60 per cent as high as it was among clerical workers. The question was whether this was because heavy labor is beneficial in promoting resistance to many acute respiratory or even some chronic illnesses, an important feature if true. But another factor had to be weighed if the conclusions of the investigation were to be accurate. Production workers were paid only for time actually worked, whereas clerical workers usually received their regular pay during short absences (Meigs 1948).

BIBLIOGRAPHY

CHEYNE, G. 1725. *An essay on health and long life.* 6th ed. London: George Strahan.

DANIEL, G. H. 1942. Social and economic conditions and the incidence of rheumatic heart disease. *J. Roy. Statist. Soc.* **105**:197–212.

DOLL, R. and AVERY-JONES, F. 1952. Occupational factors in the aetiology of gastric and duodenal ulcers. *Spec. Rept. Ser. No. 276.* London: Medical Research Council.

GAFAFER, W. M. 1943. Sickness absenteeism among male and female industrial workers, 1933–42 inclusive. *Public Health Rept.* **58:**1250–54.

GREENWOOD, M. 1948. *Some British pioneers of social medicine.* London: Oxford University Press.

HAMILTON, A. 1943. *Exploring the dangerous trades; the autobiography of Alice Hamilton, M.D.* Boston: Little, Brown & Co.

MEIGS, J. W. 1948. Illness and injury rates in small industrial plants. *Occupational Med.* **5:**11–23.

MORRIS, J. N. 1964. *Uses of epidemiology.* 2d ed. Edinburgh: E. & S. Livingstone.

PAUL, J. R. 1949. Poliomyelitis attack rates in American troops 1940–1948. *Am. J. Hyg.* **50:**57–62.

REED, L. J. 1949. Principles applying to the collection of information on health as related to socio-environmental factors. In *Backgrounds of social medicine.* New York: Milbank Memorial Fund.

REID, D. D. 1954. Statistical and epidemiological methods in occupational medicine. In *Industrial medicine and hygiene.* London: Butterworth & Co.

RYLE, J. 1948. *Changing disciplines: lectures on the history, method and motives of social pathology.* London, New York: Oxford University Press.

STEWART, A. and HUGHES, J. P. W. 1949. Tuberculosis in industry: An epidemiologic study. *Brit. Med. J.* 1926–29. **1:**926

———. 1951. Mass radiography findings in the Northamptonshire boot and shoe industry, 1945–46. *Ibid.* pp. 899–906.

VIETS, H. R. 1949. George Cheyne, 1673–1743. *Bull. Hist. Med.* **23:**435–52.

PART III

Sample Diseases

CHAPTER XV

Rheumatic Fever

Rheumatic fever cannot be considerd a true infectious disease. It is related to a true infection or, more accurately, is the occasional late (presumably allergic) response to a Group A hemolytic streptococcal infection and thus merits the designation of what Greenwood (1935) has called a "crowd disease," that is, a disease spread through close contact between persons. Although rheumatic fever does have certain features of a delayed allergic response following infection, I believe that this disease, which has for so long been considered separately, should be included today under the general heading of Group A streptococcal infections. From the standpoint of a taxonomist, I would assume the role of a "lumper" rather than a "splitter," for it is difficult for me to assume that the epidemiology of rheumatic fever and Group A streptococcal infections are fundamentally different. This latter point of view has been taken by many expert students of "both" diseases.

Historically, it is hard to know just where to begin the story of rheumatic fever. As long as it was a disease in which acute arthritis was the only identifying sign, it was indistinguishable from other acute and chronic arthritides, so that little can be said about its existence prior to the nineteenth century.

That heart disease was part of the clinical picture of rheumatic fever did not come to light until about 1800. Pitcairn and Jenner (Coombs 1924) in England both spoke about the significance of the relationship. This concept gave rheumatic fever some degree of individuality, but it did not become a well-established entity until about 1850, when through the work of Bouillaud and later Trousseau in France, the juvenile forms began to be recognized.

The possibility that rheumatic fever might result from upper respiratory infection developed toward the end of the century in England. The concept was based on observations by Haig-Brown in 1886 and, later, by others on a sequential relationship between tonsillitis and rheumatic fever. As tonsillitis gradually was recognized as an integral part of the clinical picture the medical profession slowly became aware of the intricacy and magnitude of the problem.

Dominant among the changing points of view held in the nineteenth and early twentieth centuries about the pathogenesis of rheumatic fever was constant reference to the idea that exposure to cold and dampness was one, if not the main, cause of the acute (or chronic) arthritis in this disease. This view is now usually attributed to the circumstance that exposure to cold and wet or an abrupt fall in barometric pressure is often immediately followed by painful joint symptoms in some chronic or subacute arthritics. Or, to choose a different line entirely, this view could have been based on the conjecture that cold, wet weather drives people in doors and thus paves the way for them to acquire more than their usual quota of hemolytic streptococcal infections, some of which in turn precipitate attacks of rheumatic fever. This latter is probably too simple an explanation.

CURRENT CONCEPTS OF THE CLINICAL PICTURE AND PATHOGENESIS

In the early 1930's, it became apparent that it was not enough to designate the events preceding an acute attack of rheumatic fever as a "tonsillar focus of infection," or even as an undifferentiated example of "upper respiratory infection." When bacteriological studies were brought to bear on these infections, the majority of them were found to be due to Group A hemolytic streptococcal infections, which in some ways act "as the detonator to an explosion of illness within the patient." Since the primary observations of Coburn (1931), Glover and Griffith (1931), and others, evidence of this has continued to accumulate, indicating that rheumatic fever is one of the non-suppurative sequelae of infections caused by various types of Group A hemolytic streptococci. Overt examples of acute manifestations of these infections include: streptococcal sore throat, acute follicular tonsillitis, scarlet fever, and otitis media. The late manifestations of these (usually pharyngeal) hemolytic streptococcal infections have long been a puzzle. Prominent among them are acute hemorrhagic nephritis and rheumatic fever. The former is more commonly induced by a few sero-types of hemolytic streptococci, the latter by many types. There is a whole spectrum of clinical patterns of illness that follow acute streptococcal illness and could go under the name of rheumatic fever, including at one end slight sore throat, mild fever, swollen lymph glands, elevated sedimentation rate, and so on. Indeed these late manifestations may be so slight as to reach the vanishing point, although they are sometimes evidences of a sensitization phenomenon which presage the patient's susceptibility to an overt attack of rheumatic fever following a subsequent acute attack of streptococcal infection. At the other end of the spectrum are those full blown symptoms and signs of rheumatic fever that fulfill the Jones' diagnostic criteria. These clinical patterns have been discussed fully by Feinstein and Spagnuolo (1962).

No more poignant evidence exists in firmly establishing the relationship between the "trigger mechanism" of an acute hemolytic streptococcal infection and rheumatic fever than that which can be drawn from clinical and serological observations and from reports of the striking effects antibiotics exert in reducing the incidence of rheumatic fever when the preceding streptococcal infection receives early treatment. The significance of early treatment was demonstrated in programs conducted to reduce recurrent attacks of rheumatic fever in cardiac homes for children through the daily prophylactic use of antibiotics. In a military population, a local reduction in the incidence of rheumatic fever was effected by the prompt and early treatment of all acute streptococcal infections (Rammelkamp *et al.* 1952); this type of prophylactic program has also proved effective in schools and small communities.

Therefore, on the basis of what might seem to be a common

etiology, the epidemiology of rheumatic fever and that of hemolytic streptococcal infections would seem to be mutually related, if not identical. Actually, however, we know precious little about the mechanisms involved in this delayed form of sensitivity in relation to many infectious diseases. It may be that these late responses to a foreign antigen come about as a result of the antigen having become fixed to the tissues. For instance, in glomerulonephritis, it has been thought that the streptococcal antigen becomes fixed to the glomeruli of the kidney and that antibodies acting against this site cause inflammation of the glomerular tissue. It takes little imagination to see how this same process might occur with a related antigen on the delicate valves of the heart.

General Prevalence

There is good reason to suspect that rheumatic fever may exist in nearly all inhabited parts of the globe. That overt forms are more prevalent in some places and during some seasons is recognized. This, of course, is true of many respiratory diseases. Estimates of rheumatic fever frequently are not completely accurate, for many of them are actually crude opinions based on clinical impressions rather than accurate measurements and were made before the Jones' diagnostic criteria were widely accepted.

This does not make the task of recording the frequency of a recurrent and chronic disease such as rheumatic fever any easier. What the epidemiologist desires to know is the number of new overt cases per year. This figure is usually beyond his reach, however. As a substitute, one can measure death rates for cases of acute active rheumatic fever or deaths among persons who have inactive rheumatic heart disease. One can measure, by survey methods, the prevalence of rheumatic heart disease in samples of school children or adults. One can measure the incidence of recognized and reported acute cases from health department records. None of these methods records the degree of ill-health for which this disease is responsible, and it is the latter feature that colors clinical impressions. By and large, however, current methods for determining the incidence or prevalence of rheumatic heart disease are much better than they used to be.

Practically all patients who die as a result of acute or subacute rheumatic fever have active rheumatic heart disease; in other words, these are cardiac deaths.[1] Most cardiac deaths that occur between the ages of five and twenty-five years are due to rheumatic fever; this feature helps the statistician, who may compute the rheumatic fever mortality data on an age-specific basis, considering only the juvenile and young adult groups. Among older people, an analysis of over-all cardiac mortality rates will reveal many examples in which early or advanced arteriosclerosis and other degenerative conditions are combined with old rheumatic heart disease. Statistically speaking, "old rheumatic heart disease" in adults of increasing age becomes more and more deeply buried under unqualified terms—arteriosclerotic heart disease, chronic fibrous myocarditis, endocarditis, and so on. Above the age of twenty-five the etiology is, therefore, more problematical; and with infantile groups (less than five years of age) it is also complicated by the fact that deaths from congenital heart disease are more prominent than at other ages. The 5–19 (or 5–24) age-specific mortality rate can be considered as a most useful index of frequency of rheumatic fever deaths.

A general over-all mortality estimate (based on data for 1939–41) derived from the 5–19 age group in the United States gives the rate as 11.7 per 100,000 per annum (see Table 4). This death rate, in the United States, England and elsewhere has nevertheless been declining (see Fig. 24) and this probably reflects a general decline in morbidity as well.

Several qualifying features condition the death rate besides age, such as race and socioeconomic status. These are of

[1] The implication of this statement is that relatively few patients die today from rheumatic fever without carditis, but when death occurs, it is due to active rheumatic heart disease. Many patients die years later with old rheumatic disease, of course, who show no clinical or morphologic evidence of "rheumatic activity," or rheumatic fever.

159

sufficient magnitude to make it difficult to compare the death rates from rheumatic fever between different countries. In the United States, however, diagnostic criteria are fairly uniform, and comparisons between geographical areas can be done. Wolff's figures, listed in Table 4, although a little out of date, have attempted this, and are informative. They have also been adjusted to compensate for the Negro population in various

TABLE 4

UNITED STATES AVERAGE ANNUAL DEATH RATES PER 100,000 FOR ACUTE
RHEUMATIC FEVER PLUS DISEASES OF THE HEART IN CHILDREN,
5–19 YEARS OF AGE, WITH SEPARATE RATES BY RACE (1939–41)

Geographic Divisions (Ranked According to Crude Rates)	Crude Death Rates (All Races)	Geographic Divisions (Ranked According to Adjusted Rates)	Adjusted Death Rates [a] (All Races)
Entire country	11.7	Entire country	11.7
1. Pacific	7.7	1. Pacific	8.3
2. West–South Central	8.8	2. West–South Central	8.4
3. West–North Central	9.3	3. East–South Central	9.6
4. East–South Central	10.2	4. South Atlantic	9.8
5. New England	10.5	5. West–North Central	9.9
6. South Atlantic	11.1	6. New England	12.0
7. East–North Central	12.4	7. East–North Central	13.3
8. Mountain	15.3	8. Mountain	15.3
9. Middle Atlantic	16.3	9. Middle Atlantic	17.4
(Ranked According to Rates for White Children)	White	(Ranked According to Rates for Non-White Children)	Non-white
Entire country	11.1	Entire country	16.6
1. Pacific	7.4	1. West–South Central	12.7
2. West–South Central	7.8	2. East–South Central	13.1
3. South Atlantic	8.9	3. Mountain	14.2
4. East–South Central	9.1	4. Pacific	14.7
5. West–North Central	9.1	5. West–North Central	16.1
6. New England	10.3	6. South Atlantic	16.4
7. East–North Central	11.9	7. East–North Central	24.1
8. Mountain	15.4	8. New England	24.9
9. Middle Atlantic	15.6	9. Middle Atlantic	30.5

[a] Adjusted for constant proportions of white and non-white children in the different geographic divisions. Data from Wolff, 1948.

sections of the country. The increased mortality rate among Negroes from this disease, as from tuberculosis, has made this necessary.

In Table 4 one observes that the highest rates are recorded in New England, the Middle Atlantic states, the Mountain states, and in the East-North Central states. This distribution points out the ecological importance of two rather divergent features: macroclimatic conditions, including those characteristic of high altitudes; and microclimatic conditions characteristic of the crowded living conditions in industrial cities or towns in the northern half of the United States.

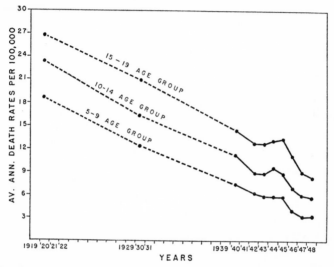

FIG. 24. Declining mortality rates for rheumatic fever and diseases of the heart during the period 1919–48 in the United States in three age groups representing the white population only. (Data from Wolff, G., 1953. The decline and variation in mortality from rheumatic heart disease in the United States. *Bull. St. Francis San.* **10**:1.)

MORBIDITY DETERMINATIONS

For various reasons rheumatic fever is poorly reported in most places. Difficulties in the diagnosis have been partially responsible (some of these have already been discussed; see also Feinstein and Spagnuolo 1962). In Scandinavia, where the reporting seems to be more accurate than elsewhere, crude incidence rates have been recorded during recent decades at 1 to 3 per 1,000 per annum. These rates are far from fixed. They vary from place to place and are subject to change with each decade. Adequate data for the United States probably do not yet exist.

There have been many surveys that have not necessarily been limited in scope to rheumatic fever but have yielded rheumatic fever rates in association with streptococcal infections in the same population. Those reported from the first national health survey conducted by the United States Public Health Service were mentioned in chapter 10, and some of the data appear in Fig. 10.

RHEUMATIC HEART DISEASE SURVEYS

Still another and more indirect method of measuring the prevalence of rheumatic fever or, more accurately, the effects of rheumatic fever lies in determining the prevalence of active and inactive rheumatic heart disease in groups of young people or adults. In the United States such heart disease surveys have been made on groups of school and college students. Both groups seem to furnish a better estimate of the situation in a given population than do surveys on workmen or military recruits, who may have had some preliminary screening. They are also between the desirable ages of 5 and 24. Data from these special cardiac surveys of American school children reveal, as one might have suspected, wide variations, ranging from rates under 5 per 1,000 in California and the Southwest to 60 per 1,000 in the Middle Atlantic states and the Mountain states of the West and Northwest.

The extensive nationwide survey Marienfeld *et al.* (1964) conducted in U.S. college freshmen in 1956–60 yields an adequate picture for the United States for that period. According to their scoring system, which included cases of rheumatic fever as well as definite and probable cases of rheumatic heart disease, their national rate was 17.5 per 1,000, a not inconsiderable rate indicating that in spite of the spectacular decline in rheumatic fever incidence in the past generation, it remains an important public health problem. Their national rate for rheumatic heart disease alone was about 5.7 per 1,000. The geographic distribution of rheumatic fever with or without rheumatic heart disease showed the highest rates in the Rocky Mountain area and in the northern temperate zone.

A recent study by Stokes and Dawber (1956) reports upon a special urban cardiac survey in adults. It was conducted on a random sampling of 4,500 people (aged 30–59) in the city of Framingham, Massachusetts, during the period 1948–53. Here the rheumatic heart disease prevalence was recorded as 27 per 1,000.

Transmission

In many ways Group A hemolytic streptococci, of which there are many serotypes, represents the seed in an epidemiological sense. It is *the* etiologic agent of rheumatic fever, but, to say it is the only etiologic factor is inadequate. The conditioning factor of the host is another aspect of etiology that assumes importance in this disease.

Acute streptococcal infections are usually acquired between the ages of one and twenty years, most frequently in the early school-age period. They are transmitted mainly through human association, probably through direct contact, and to a lesser extent indirectly through the medium of contaminated objects such as food or milk (see Fig. 12). Carriers are prevalent in the population and are especially numerous among children, who may be largely responsible for the dissemination of these infections.

AGE AND SUSCEPTIBILITY

The difficulty of differentiating between first and subsequent attacks of rheumatic fever has been responsible for divergent views about its actual incidence by age. In its familiar forms, however, first attacks of clinically recognizable rheumatic fever occur largely during school age. They are rare in infants under two years and not common under four years. This emphasizes how age conditions susceptibility. The infant apparently must grow up to become "rheumatic," and regardless of close exposure he usually succeeds in reaching the age of six before the disease is acquired in recognizable clinical forms. This does not mean that the groundwork of the "sensitization phenomena" is not being laid in the years preceding the age of six, which may indeed be important years for conditioning the potential patient for subsequent acquisition of this illness but it is after the age of five that the Jones' diagnostic criteria becomes readily applicable. Probably each child acquires his quota of streptococcal infections (either apparent or inapparent) from an unknown number of serotypes of streptococci, particularly during his early years in school, and from each of these infections he runs a slight risk of acquiring rheumatic fever—or a greater risk of reactivating his case of rheumatic fever if he is susceptible and not under prophylaxis.

Susceptibility to both first and recurrent attacks decline in the years after puberty. But from the clinical standpoint rheumatic fever cannot be regarded solely as a disease of childhood, for primary attacks predispose the individual to recurrent attacks, and active rheumatic carditis and polyarthritis are common enough during adolescence and young adult life.

A certain amount of resistance to Group A hemolytic streptococcal infections seems to be gained, perhaps as a result of heterologous immunity, after adolescence. And yet these infections are common enough in military camps. But at least the incidence curve of age-specific, overt cases of tonsillitis, the great majority of which are presumably streptococcal in origin, declines in the age group 15–25 (See Fig. 10). But there is a difference of opinion here, for according to Johnson *et al.* (1964), who observed a documented group of adolescents and adults, the rate of overt cases of streptococcal infection was not significantly different in the two groups; it was the incidence of a symptomatic infection that accounted for the gradient.

Rammelkamp *et al.* (1952a) observed in adults in a military population that approximately 3 per cent of overt, streptococcal infections of the respiratory tract were complicated by frank rheumatic fever. Estimates of this kind have been made by many. Of course, if one includes subclinical streptococcal infections, this might bring the ratio down far lower than even 1.0 per cent.

SEX

Except in the case of Sydenham's chorea,[2] the influence of sex on rheumatic fever is not profound. In childhood groups below the age of 13 rheumatic fever is more likely to develop in girls than in boys, owing perhaps to the fact that chorea is more common in girls. In adolescence and adult life, active rheumatic fever is more likely to develop in males than in females. This does not hold true for Negroes, for females seem to be particularly vulnerable during the childbearing period, to severe rheumatic fever with an increased death rate (see Fig. 19).

RACIAL SUSCEPTIBILITY

It is not certain whether race influences susceptibility or resistance, and data on this point are apt to be unreliable and conflicting. The case mortality rate in the Negro is higher in the United States than in the white, although the over-all incidence of rheumatic fever among negroes and whites is about equal.

ANTHROPOLOGICAL TYPES

Many investigators believe that certain types of human physique carry with them a special susceptibility for the development of rheumatic fever, but here again data regarding these views are somewhat conflicting.

FAMILIAL INCIDENCE

A voluminous literature bears witness to the fact that the prevalence of rheumatic fever and rheumatic heart disease is high in certain families. It has been shown, for instance, that in families in which the parents have suffered from rheumatic fever, the prevalence of this disease is more than twice as high as in other families. Also, in so-called "rheumatic" families, 8 to 10 per cent of exposed persons are involved, in contrast to 2.9 per cent in the families of healthy controls. This is similar to the familial incidence of tuberculosis. An illustration of a family tree appears

[2] A nervous disorder, also known as St. Vitus' dance, that is generally included in the spectrum of post-streptococal inflammation.

in Fig. 25. Pickles (1943) observed five generations of this family and recorded his findings.

Favoring the importance of hereditary factors, Wilson and Schweitzer (1954) have reaffirmed their previous conclusion that susceptibility to rheumatic fever is inherited as a simple recessive trait. They also pointed out that the demonstration of hereditary susceptibility does not exclude the operation of environmental factors. Gray, Quinn, and Quinn (1952) reached essentially this same conclusion in their study, but placed more emphasis on the

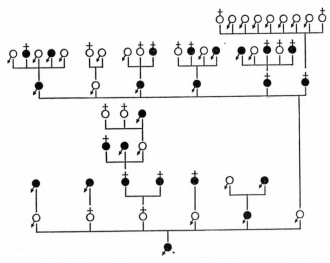

FIG. 25. Dr. Pickles' "rheumatic family" with a record covering five generations. Black circles indicate members of the family with a history of rheumatic fever or signs of mitral stenosis. The spouses (or in-laws) are not recorded, and it is stated that in no instance was the spouse rheumatic, so the story is uncomplicated in this respect. (Data from Pickles, W. N., 1943. A rheumatic family. *Lancet* 2:241.)

environment. Others have agreed that inheritance may play a major role in determining familial aggregation of cases, but a Mendelian mechanism has not been established. Still others doubt that familial prevalence is due to anything other than environmental factors that facilitate the opportunities for exposure to hemolytic streptococci. This clustering of cases through several generations requires much more study in the fields of human genetics and clinical epidemiology.

The rheumatic family, in which more than one case of rheumatic fever or rheumatic heart disease has been detected, is familiar enough to general practitioners of medicine and to pediatricians. By examining all members of a given family when a case of rheumatic fever is discovered and by questioning and examining the parents in particular about symptoms and signs, as one might do in a tuberculosis case, one often obtains information of clinical epidemiologic significance.

A record of events sketched on a family chart is of advantage here, and several examples of such charts have already been shown (Figs. 4, 11).[3] This intimate study of the family group can demonstrate the pattern of spread of streptococcal infections and rheumatic fever through household populations. In the example given here (Fig. 26) each vertical line indicates a member of the family, the length of the line being equal to the age of the individual in 1955. There was clinical evidence of streptococcal infection in the early years of the life of the juvenile members, but signs suggesting rheumatic fever did not appear in the first child until the age of eight years; in the second child, possibly at five but definitely at ten years; and in the third, at thirteen years. Two possible patterns of spread of the rheumatic fever symptoms are indicated by the arrows *A* and *B*. *A* is the explosive spread common to acute clinical infections. This is the way a wave of acute streptococcal illness will sweep through a family, but it is unusual for this type of spread to occur with first attacks of rheumatic fever in a family. The oblique or sequential spread, indicated by *B* or *B*[1], is more apt to occur. This may indicate that the trigger mechanism of the infection is constantly present or continually recurring; but not until each susceptible child reaches the age of six or eight will he develop recognizable symptoms of rheumatic fever for the first time.

IMMUNITY

As previously mentioned, it takes factors other than the seed, that is, more than streptococci, to produce a case of rheumatic fever, and even though Group A streptococci may be present in a

[3] Such charts have been employed since 1930 at the New Haven Hospital, sometimes as part of the hospital record.

community and conditions may be favorable for their spread, very few cases of rheumatic fever will result unless susceptible hosts are also present in adequate numbers. Stollerman (1956) has shown that rheumatic fever does not recur unless a strepto-

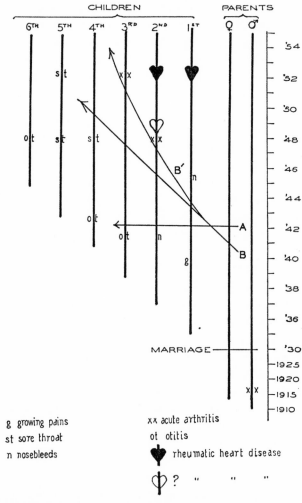

Fig. 26. Schematic diagram of a family in which there are six children, in three of whom the diagnosis of rheumatic fever and/or rheumatic heart disease has been made. (From Paul, J. R., 1957. *The epidemiology of rheumatic fever.* 3d ed. New York: American Heart Association.)

coccal infection associated with a detectable immunologic response occurs. There are a variety of methods for measuring serologically the immunologic responses to Group A streptococcal infections. The most common test is anti-streptolysin O (ASLO), but there are several more. Nearly all investigators record high values immediately after a streptococcal infection, but these high levels are apt to be more or less temporary. Moderate levels usually persist during adulthood with some decline in titer in old age. As for the usual ASLO responses in patients who have had one or more attacks of rheumatic fever, these produces high levels which remain high and last longer than in non-rheumatics.

Many attempts have been made, notably with ASLO tests, to outline the geographical distribution of cases of streptococcal infections or rheumatic fever by serologic methods. These attempts have been disappointing for the most part, and it is difficult to know why.

What is the conditioning factor in the host that makes a small percentage of those infected with Group A hemolytic streptococci develop rheumatic fever while another group fails to develop such complications? This crucial question makes us wonder again whether the potential rheumatic patient is born with the capacity for reacting with a special "rheumatic response" to upper respiratory streptococcal infections, or whether he develops this capacity because he has acquired more than his share of multiple infections with heterologous types of streptococci early in life. Though individuals can acquire multiple sequential infections for the numerous serotypes of streptococci, once infection has been induced for any one type, permanent homologous immunity apparently results.

CLIMATE AND ENVIRONMENT

The rate of exposure to these streptococci, yielding as it does marked seasonal upswings, may differ enormously in different places and from year to year in the same place. An excellent example of the variation in rates in a single community is provided by a study carried on under natural conditions in

Holland with a population of about 5,000 (Valkenburg *et al.* 1963). During the two-year period in which the survey was conducted, only 233 patients representing overt cases out of the whole population were referred into the study. From them 151 strains of Group A hemolytic streptococci were isolated, indicating a documented rate of 1.5 per cent of cases. As in other surveys the per cent of inapparent infections was extensive, and it was the authors' belief that the referred cases barely represented 10 per cent of the infections which had actually occurred in this population during the two years; a village rate of perhaps 11.2 per cent would have been more realistic. During the two-year period, 10 different streptococcal serotypes were found circulating in the village population. Fortunately virtually all strains were typable; only one type (type 1) showed an epidemic increase; other types (12 and 14) were continuously present; 69 per cent of all cases were caused by four types. The authors felt justified in assuming that in the Netherlands, at least, every person has had 7 or 8 infections of different streptococcal types before the age of fifty.

Two characteristics that have long captured the imagination of students of rheumatic fever are its tendency to flourish (*a*) in cold damp climates and often at high altitudes, such as in Colorado or Mexico City, and (*b*) under crowded urban conditions, such as in the slums of London or New York. But not much is known about the true difference in incidence of rheumatic fever in temperate versus tropical areas or in wet versus arid areas of the world.

Reference has already been made earlier in this chapter (Table 4) to the high rheumatic fever mortality rates in two geographical districts—in the Mountain states and in states where industrial cities predominate. The observations on college students reported by Marienfeld *et al.* (1964) also mention the Rocky Mountain area and the northern temperate zone. This partially reflects the fact that cold damp weather promotes the spread of upper respiratory infections. In other words, streptococcal infections and rheumatic fever automatically follow a parallel seasonal trend. Naturally this trend differs in different localities, but the number of acute attacks of rheumatic fever in the eastern United States reaches a maximum incidence during late winter and early spring (see Fig. 27). Cold weather in itself

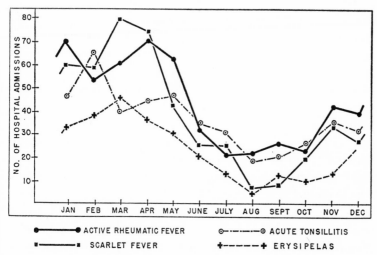

Fig. 27. Seasonal occurrence of the onset of hospitalized cases of rheumatic fever and three streptococcal diseases in New Haven County, covering the period 1929–38. The rheumatic fever series consists of 526 cases, the scarlet fever, of 458, the acute tonsillitis, of 443, and the erysipelas, of 285. (From Paul, J. R. [ed.], 1943. *The epidemiology of rheumatic fever.* 2d ed. New York: Metropolitan Life Insurance Co.)

does not seem to be sufficient; but cold, coupled with dampness, particularly in situations which promote crowding indoors, seem to represent the predisposing conditions.

SOCIAL AND LIVING CONDITIONS

Rheumatic fever was originally branded in England as a "social disease" because its highest incidence was among the poorer children of industrial towns. This also has implicated the various factors we have just discussed—exposure to cold and dampness and bad living conditions such as poor housing, crowding, and perhaps malnutrition. These factors do not receive the same emphasis today as they did in the 1920's because the incidence of the disease in England and the United States has

171

declined so much and because urban living conditions have improved mightily in both these countries during the past two decades.

Nevertheless, the effect of socioeconomic conditions on the prevalence of rheumatic heart disease in the United States can still be demonstrated. An urban study by Quinn and Quinn (1951) indicates that the mortality rates due to rheumatic heart disease in the city of New Haven, estimated during the years 1920–48, have been consistently higher among people living in the poorest areas than among those in the better areas. Their findings confirm, in general, reports from England by Knowelden (1949), who noted a moderate degree of association between the death rate due to rheumatic heart disease and its higher proportion in employed males belonging to the lowest social classes.

The broad concept that poverty and all its attendant conditions are associated with an increased incidence of rheumatic fever finds considerable basis in the results reported by Collins in 1947 from a nationwide survey dating from the 1930's in the United States. Family income rates were computed for white persons in a large number of cities. It was found that as the economic status fell, the incidence rates for new cases of rheumatic fever, chorea, and rheumatic heart disease rose rather consistently, as did the prevalence rates for disability (see Fig. 28). The rates of families on relief stand out exceptionally high in this illustration, a feature which might be explained because the presence of a chronically ill child in the family may be why some of these families sought and received relief.

Poverty often brings with it a poor microclimate and many of its component features, to which reference has been made in the differential analysis by Daniels (see Table 3). One of these interrelated features is poor housing, which may be dependent on building construction as well as on soil and drainage facilities. This in turn points up the supposed relationship of rheumatic fever with dampness. It would be difficult to evaluate these implications unless one knew whether or not the concentration of rheumatic fever cases along water courses merely reflected the fact that this was the site of the cheapest houses. On the other hand, it is common knowledge (although not well established on a scientific basis) that damp or wet living quarters do tend to promote the spread of upper respiratory infections. Presumably these same living conditions tend to spread hemolytic streptococc-

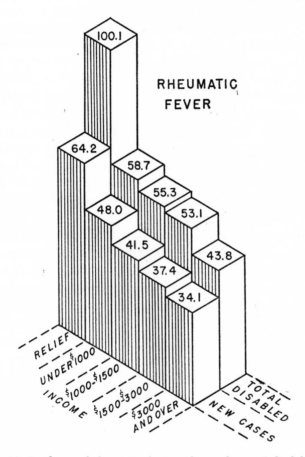

FIG. 28. Incidence of rheumatic fever and prevalence of disability per 100,000 in children, 5–19 years of age among white families of different income levels in 84 cities and towns in 19 states during the 1930's. (Data from Collins, 1947. Public Health Reports, Suppl. No. 198.)

cal infections as well as other upper respiratory infections, but whether the exposure of young children to such conditions promotes rheumatic fever is unknown. It is obvious that many more controlled epidemiologic observations are needed before

173

the relationship of rheumatic fever to dampness can be regarded as proved or understandable.

Crowding, poverty, and malnutrition go together; the situation is full of interdependent contingencies, including family size. Since the early observations of Perry and Roberts in England (1937) established a direct relationship between the degree of crowding and the incidence of rheumatic fever, the living-space factor has received increasing attention (see Table 3). In the United States, rheumatic heart disease is still acquired at a higher rate among school children living in urban rather than in rural areas. The unfavorable effect of crowding in a home is supported by the long-term observations on a group of forty rheumatic and thirty non-rheumatic families by Gray *et al.* (1952). It is believed that crowding in the home may facilitate the spread and maintenance of many infections within the family circle; its effect upon the prevalence of tuberculosis and pneumonia is recognized. According to one theory about rheumatic fever, crowding in the home particularly among young children, promotes repeated infection due to different types of streptococci and thus induces the occurrence of the rheumatic state. Within a little cosmos of very susceptible hosts, one infection can come fast upon the heels of another at an age when the child is poorly fitted to handle the situation. Here is another field that calls for more investigation.

BIBLIOGRAPHY

COBURN, A. F. 1931. *Factor of infection in the rheumatic state.* Baltimore: Williams & Wilkins Co.

COOMBS, C. F. 1924. *Rheumatic heart disease.* Bristol: John Wright & Sons, Ltd.

DANIELS, G. H. 1942. Social and economic conditions and the incidence of rheumatic heart disease. *J. Roy. Statist. Soc.* **105**:170.

FEINSTEIN, R. and SPAGNUOLO, M. 1962. The clinical patterns of acute rheumatic fever: a reappraisal. *Medicine* **41**:279–305.

GLOVER, J. A., and GRIFFITH, F. 1931. Acute tonsillitus and some of its sequels: Epidemiological and bacteriological observations. *Brit. Med. J.* **2**:521.

GRAY, F. G., QUINN, R. W., and QUINN, J. P. 1952. A long-term survey of rheumatic and non-rheumatic families; with particular reference to environment and heredity. *Am. J. Med.* 13:400.

HAIG-BROWN, C. 1886. *Tonsillitis in adolescents.* London: Bailliere, Tindal, and Cox.

JOHNSON, E. E., STOLLERMAN, G. H. and GROSSMAN, B. J. 1964. Rheumatic recurrences in patients not receiving continuous prophylaxis. *J.A.M.A.* 190:407–13.

KNOWELDEN, J. 1949. Mortality from rheumatic heart disease in children and young adults in England and Wales. *Brit. J. Soc. Med.* 3:29.

MADSEN, T. and KALBAK, K. 1940. Investigations on rheumatic fever subsequent to epidemics of septic sore throat (especially milk epidemics). *Acta Path. Microbiol. Scand.* 17:305.

MARIENFELD, C. J., ROBINS, M., SANDIDGE, R. P. and FINDLAN, C. 1964. Rheumatic fever and rheumatic heart disease among U.S. college freshmen, 1956–60. *Public Health Repts.* 79:789–811.

PAUL, J. R. 1941. *Rheumatic fever in New Haven.* Lancaster, Pa.: Science Press.

———. (ed). 1943. *Epidemiology of rheumatic fever and some of its public health aspects.* 2d ed. New York: Metropolitan Life Insurance Co.

———. 1957. *The epidemiology of rheumatic fever.* 3d ed. New York: American Heart Association.

PAUL, J. R., and SALINGER, R. 1931. The spread of rheumatic fever through families. *J. Clin. Invest.* 10:33.

PERRY, C. B. and ROBERTS, J. A. F. 1937. Study on the variability in the incidence of rheumatic heart disease within the city of Bristol. *Brit. Med. J.* 2:154.

PICKLES, W. N. 1943. A rheumatic family. *Lancet* 2:241.

QUINN, R. W. and MARTIN, M. P. 1961. Natural occurrence of hemolytic streptococci in school children: five-year study. *Am. J. Hyg.* 73:193–208.

QUINN, R. W. and QUINN, J. P. 1951. Mortality due to rheumatic heart disease in the socio-economic districts of New Haven, Connecticut. *Yale J. Biol. Med.* 24:15.

RAMMELKAMP, C. H., DENNY, F. W., and WANNAMAKER, L. W. 1952. (*a*) Studies on the epidemiology of rheumatic fever in the Armed Services. In: *Rheumatic fever: A symposium.* L. THOMAS (ed.). Minneapolis: University of Minnesota Press.

RAMMELKAMP, C. H., HOUSER, H. B., HAHN, E. O., WANNAMAKER, L. W., DENNY, F. W., and ECKHARDT, G. C. 1952. The prevention of rheumatic fever. In *Rheumatic fever: A sympo-*

sium, L. Thomas. (ed.). Minneapolis: University of Minnesota Press.

Rantz, L. A., Maroney, M., and Dicaprio, J. M. 1951. Antistreptolysin O response following hemolytic streptococcus infection in early childhood. *Arch. Intern. Med.* **87**:360.

Raska, K. 1960. Epidemiology of streptococcal infections and their sequelae. Presented at WHO Symposium on laboratory and epidemiological studies of streptococcal infections in Central Europe. Prague, December 6–10, 1960.

Siegel, A. C., Johnson, E. E. and Stollerman, G. H. 1961. Controlled studies of streptococcal pharyngitis in pediatric population. I. Factors related to attack rate of rheumatic fever. *New Engl. J. Med.* **265**:559–66.

Stokes, J. and Dawber, T. R. 1956. Rheumatic heart disease in the Framingham study. *New Engl. J. Med.* **255**:1228.

Stollerman, G. H. 1956. Relationship of immune response to group A streptococci to course of acute, chronic and recurrent rheumatic fever. *Am. J. Med.* **20**:163.

Wilson, M. G. and Schweitzer, M. D. 1954. Pattern of hereditary susceptibility in rheumatic fever. *Circulation* **10**:699.

Wolff, 1948. Childhood mortality from rheumatic fever and rheumatic heart disease. Publication No. 322. Washington, D.C.: Department of Health, Education, and Welfare, Children's Bureau.

Valkenburg, H. A., Goslings, W. R. O., Bots, A. W., DeMoor, C. E., and Lorrier, J. C. 1963. Attack rate of streptococcal pharyngitis, rheumatic fever and glomerulonephritis in the general population. II. The epidemiology of streptococcal pharyngitis in one village during a two-year period. *New Eng. J. Med.* **268**:694–701.

Poliomyelitis

From the standpoint of its epidemiology, few diseases, infectious or otherwise, have received more attention in the past than poliomyelitis. Because of the mass of information that is available today, this chapter can be only the briefest kind of abridgment. Perhaps one can afford to be brief because interest in this infection has already begun to wane. Since the time the first inactivated vaccine was introduced in 1955 (Salk 1955), the incidence of poliomyelitis has declined. The spectacular reduction of the incidence of poliomyelitis wrought in those countries where the inactivated and the attenuated poliovirus vaccines have been used efficiently has been little short of miraculous. From a maximum of about 40,000 cases a year in the United States the total dropped to 120 cases recorded in 1964! Small wonder that most people feel that this is not only a cause for rejoicing but for putting that disease out of their mind. Most would be just as happy if they never heard about "polio" again, except as a bit of history.

And yet, in spite of this sudden and understandable decline of general interest in poliomyelitis, few diseases can be studied to better advantage today. The use of attenuated strains of poliovirus in vaccine trials has opened up all sorts of channels for a new kind of exploration and exploitation of human experimental epidemiology (Sabin 1962). Perhaps similar studies on live attenuated strains of measles virus vaccine could soon follow suit. These investigations give promise of determining portals of entrance or exit of the virus, the circumstances under which dissemination is most likely to occur, and the solutions to a host of other problems unsolved previously because of the lack of adequate methods.

HISTORY

Infantile paralysis is probably as old as written history, but as a clinical entity it does not seem to have attracted the attention of physicians until the late eighteenth century. Clinical descriptions of it began to appear then and later from several areas: England in 1795, Italy in 1813, and India in 1823. The disease was regarded at that time as ubiquitous. Not only were there no accounts of large epidemics, but there was no mention of anything suggesting contagion, nor was the condition regarded as a medical problem of any magnitude. How prevalent poliomyelitis was later, during the greater part of the nineteenth century, is a matter of speculation, but Jacob Heine of Cannstatt, Germany, was able to collect in 1840 a considerable series of late paralytic cases. Coincidentally, North American surgeons in the 1830's made occasional mention of acute paralysis in infancy, without comment as to rarity. Apparently, the general situation in the mid-nineteenth century was reminiscent of that found today in certain tropical countries and in urban (unvaccinated) populations where substandard sanitary conditions exist, where the acute disease is endemic and limited to infants, and where it is not regarded as a problem of major importance.

The first report of what might be called an epidemic came in 1836 from Sir Charles Bell, the anatomist. He stated that a group of cases of paralysis in children had occurred in a relatively isolated community on the island of St. Helena. Bell believed that the situation "deserved looking into." In the same year Badham in England described four simultaneous cases of acute paralysis in the small community of Worksop. He, too, regarded this situation as ominous. A few years later, in 1843, a brief report by Colmer from Louisiana mentioned a group of eight to ten cases, all in infants under two years of age. But in spite of these limited and scattered outbreaks in the mid-nineteenth century, poliomyelitis was not destined to become recognized quickly as a disease entity with infectious or epidemic potentialities. Not until

1868, when fourteen cases were reported in Norway, and later, when Cordier described outbreaks in France (1888) and Medin noted others in Sweden (1891), did the medical profession begin to take the epidemic character of poliomyelitis seriously. After about 1900, epidemics of this disease appeared in northern Europe, North America, and elsewhere with ever increasing rapidity. From a comparative curiosity, infantile paralysis had turned into a scourge.

Early in the 1900's, Wickman (1911) in Sweden (whose classic work was done before the discovery of poliomyelitis virus) laid the basis for modern epidemiological concepts of this disease, placing emphasis on its infectious nature, its spread through human contact, and the importance of mild cases as carriers. The discovery of the causative virus in 1908 by Landsteiner and Popper in Vienna opened up new vistas, although for many years the path was narrow and tortuous and progress was slow until Enders *et al.* (1949) brought tissue culture methods into this field. The separation of poliovirus into three distinct serotypes was achieved in the late 1940's; the development of practical tests for the isolation of the virus from clinical cases and carriers and for determining antibodies in the early 1950's. Salk's inactivated vaccine was introduced in 1955 and the attenuated vaccines, of which Sabin's has been the most prominent, by the early 1960's.

EPIDEMIC EVOLUTION

Once the pattern of periodic epidemics within a population has been started, it is usually irreversible. Areas and approximate dates of the beginning of this transition from endemic to epidemic poliomyelitis are: Norway, 1868; Sweden, 1880; parts of western Europe in the 1880's or 1890's; the northeastern section of the United States in the 1890's; and the southeastern section about 1910. More recently, since about 1930, this epidemic evolution has affected tropical and semitropical islands such as Puerto Rico, Jamaica, Malta and Mauritius where poliomyelitis had previously been unknown or regarded as sporadic or even as extremely rare. But an unpleasant reminder that the virus was actually there all the time was the fact that the disease regularly came to the surface when visitors or groups of foreigners, such as soldiers, entered the country as "susceptible immigrants" and acquired poliomyelitis there, at far higher rates than would have been expected for that age group in their homelands. This was noted by Hillman in the Philippine Islands as early as 1936, and it happened often during World War II in both the Far East and Middle East. It has even been said that poliomyelitis is fundamentally an endemic tropical disease that strays periodically into southern or northern temperate zones. This is probably an oversimplification of a complex ecologic problem that is urgently in need of further study.

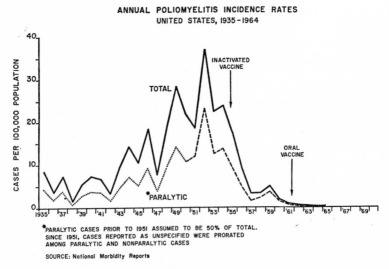

FIG. 29. Annual poliomyelitis incidence rates, United States, 1935–65. (Data from Poliomyelitis Surveillance Reports, U.S. Public Health Service, Atlanta, Ga.)

When periodic epidemics of poliomyelitis have begun to appear among the local inhabitants of a given region, a gradual or sharp increase in the average annual number of cases (as measured over ten-year periods) has usually taken place. In some countries the annual number of cases has continued to rise, as it did in the United States until 1955 when the inactivated vaccine was introduced (Fig. 29). In others the number of cases has remained at fairly high levels during 1900–1950 with irregular swings or with recurrent epidemics that may have a rough periodicity.

The world history of poliomyelitis indicates that the pattern of evolution of the disease has been experienced successively in many different areas since the late nineteenth century, and that the emergence of first epidemics is still continuing, particularly in tropical and semitropical countries (Gear 1955; Sabin 1963). The introduction of new and virulent strains of virus may have been responsible for the shift in epidemic behavior. Gear in 1948 proposed such a mechanism as an explanation for the sudden appearance in the 1940's of epidemic paralytic poliomyelitis in Africa. Presumably increased travel with correspondingly increased opportunities for the dissemination of virulent strains may have been important influences in the recent emergence of epidemic poliomyelitis in the tropics.

AGE DISTRIBUTION

Another and related type of evolution, which took place in the pre-vaccinal era and which followed or accompanied the advent of periodic epidemics, has been a gradual shift in age incidence with the majority of cases shifting from infants to children of school age or even adolescents. This feature has made the old name of infantile paralysis not as descriptive today as it once was. This shift has been in keeping with the behavior of a number of other acute, infectious, childhood diseases. It has much to do with changing ways of life in the twentieth century, particularly in the mid-twentieth century, that reflect the greater efforts made today to protect young infants from early exposure to infectious diseases than a generation or two ago. This behavior is not completely understood, but abundant evidence indicates that shifting patterns of acquired immunity in different age groups associated with changing environmental conditions such as sanitation, degree of crowding, and family size, are pertinent factors. During the pre-epidemic era fifty or sixty years ago, maximum attack rates were nearly always recorded in the infant

181

age group, a situation still common today in certain parts of the world where sanitation is substandard such as in North Africa and in some of the cities in the Middle East. But with the onset of the epidemic era in northern Europe, North America, and Australia, "infantile paralysis" became "school-child paralysis" with a shift in age incidence to the 5–9 age group. In Sweden in the days before vaccination, the ages had risen to include many young adults (Olin 1952).

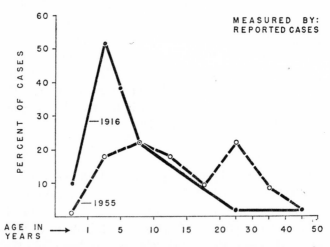

Fig. 30. Comparison of age distribution of cases of poliomyelitis in Connecticut in 1916 (continuous line) and 1955 (broken line). (Data from James C. Hart and Mila E. Rindge, Bureau of Preventable Diseases, Connecticut State Department of Health.)

How different the age distribution of cases can be within the same limited geographic area when compared at an interval of some forty years is illustrated in Fig. 30. In the northeastern part of the United States, just prior to the widespread use of the Salk vaccine, as many as 30 to 40 per cent of the patients were 15 years or older.

The two trends—a rising rate in the ten-year average annual incidence of cases and an increase in the age of the patients—are probably related. One of the explanations is that when the

182

disease is restricted to the infantile age group (0–2 years) it is milder and less apt to be recognized or reported. Thus, more than 99 per cent of infantile infections with poliovirus are inapparent infections. On the other hand, when school children represent the most susceptible age, this percentage of inapparent cases may fall well below 95 per cent. As with certain other virus diseases of children, the likelihood of acquiring the infection after the age of 7 or 8 decreases yearly, but those adolescents and adults who do become infected are harder hit. Thus severity and, correspondingly, ease of clinical recognition of the disease increases as the age of the patient progresses from 2 to 40 years. Adult cases are apt to be particularly severe. For these reasons alone, one can see how the adolescent and adult forms of the paralytic disease has seemed to increase the recorded number of cases. They attract more attention, more alarm than do an equal number of patients suffering from the milder infantile disease, many of whose symptoms may reach the vanishing point and thus may never be reported. All these percentages on age distribution concern the prevaccinal era only.

INFLUENCE OF SANITATION

The epidemiology of poliomyelitis is markedly influenced by the nature of the sanitary environment. In unvaccinated populations living under poor conditions of sanitation and hygiene, serologic surveys have shown that polioviruses are widely disseminated; infections, mostly inapparent, occur at an early age; and close to 100 per cent of the children acquire antibodies within the first few years of life (Paul *et al.* 1952). This results in a highly immune population in which only the youngest children are susceptible, paralytic cases are limited to this youngest age group, and in which epidemics are almost unknown. In contrast, in areas with high standards of living, exposure and infection are delayed until later in life; large segments of the juvenile population remain susceptible; and severe epidemics involving older children and young adults may occur when virulent strains are introduced—unless vaccination is introduced. The inverse relationship between infant mortality and the incidence of poliomyelitis also reflects a close tie between epidemics and social and sanitary conditions. When the latter improve, and infant mortality rates fall to 70–80/1,000, experience has shown that first epidemics are likely to follow within a few years (Payne 1955, Paul 1958).

GEOGRAPHICAL DISTRIBUTION

Today poliomyelitis is practically worldwide in distribution, and there is no reason to doubt that it will penetrate to every part of the inhabited globe. It has varied in different places, from extreme endemicity to severe recurrent or periodic epidemics. The wide-scale use of artificial immunization has affected its recorded incidence greatly.

CLIMATE AND SEASON

The effect of climate and season on the epidemiology of poliomyelitis is profound, but curiously enough it is poorly understood. In tropical areas, inapparent infections and paralytic cases occur more or less evenly throughout the year with only a slight concentration of cases in the hottest months. But in northern and southern temperate climates, marked seasonal variations are noted in the occurrence of inapparent infections and in clinical cases, both in years of endemic and epidemic prevalence. No satisfactory reason has yet been given to explain the summer incidence of poliomyelitis, particularly why this effect should be so sharp and dramatic. Why epidemics occur at such a higher rate during summer and early autumn in a disease obviously spread by human contact remains something of a mystery. Some factor, conditioned by summer weather—and poorly understood at present—must introduce large amounts of poliovirus into the community at certain times. The idea that human susceptibility sinks to low levels at certain times is less tenable. Meterological factors other than temperature, such as humidity and rainfall, have been investigated but no consistent correlation between these influences and the prevalence of poliomyelitis has been established.

SEX DISTRIBUTION

Like many other childhood diseases, there is relatively little difference in incidence between boys and girls. In several groups of adult cases (18 to 30 years of age) in the United States, women have acquired poliomyelitis at a higher rate than men, probably because young mothers are more heavily exposed in the home than are young fathers.

POLIOVIRUSES

Few viruses responsible for disease in man have been studied as intensively as the three known types of polioviruses. It is not necessary to go into a detailed description of these agents here.[1] Suffice it to say with regard to properties of polioviruses that it has become customary to classify the three serotypes of polioviruses, along with a much larger group known as *enteroviruses*. These include Coxsackie and Echo viruses, a large family that shares the common properties of small size (they rank among the smallest of viruses) and resistance to certain chemicals known to destroy other viruses such as ether. They grow well in tissue cultures and give rise there to cytopathogenic effects of appropriate cells (Enders *et al.* 1949). Experimental infections have a narrow host range in comparison to some of the other so-called neurotropic viruses, the family of primates being the best known example of susceptible hosts.

The poliovirus family is composed of three serotypes, (I, II, and III) of which Type I is responsible for the great majority of the cases in most parts of the world. Immunity to either a paralytic or inapparent infection, which is caused by one type of poliovirus, may protect monkeys from a paralytic reinfection with the same type of poliovirus (homotypic) but does not ordinarily protect them from infection with a heterotypic virus. Homotypic

[1] One of the best known sources of information here is the article on poliomyelitis by Dorothy M. Horstmann and David Bodian in *Viral and Rickettsial Infections of Man*, eds. Horsfall and Tamm (5th ed., Philadelphia: J. B. Lippincott and Co. 1965). An extensive bibliography accompanies this article.

paralytic reinfections are probably rare in man. With the Sabin attenuated vaccine strains, second homotypic infections can occur in 10 to 15 per cent of persons six or eight weeks after they have received live vaccine. Such reinfections are nearly always inapparent.

MODES OF SPREAD: HUMAN CONTACT

It is more or less generally accepted today that poliomyelitis is a highly infectious disease, spread largely by human association or contact. The wavelike peripheral advance of epidemics of poliomyelitis from a central focus is consistent with this theory. Unlike certain contact or crowd diseases, such as measles, in which the disease passes from one recognized case to another, the spread of poliomyelitis often occurs through the medium of mild or subclinical cases, many of which are so slight that their chance of recognition is almost nil. Nevertheless, they can nearly always be identified by virus isolation and a demonstrated rise in antibodies. In some epidemics the percentage of abortive or questionable cases is far greater than in others—a notable example was the New England epidemic of 1931 (Paul and Trask 1932).

Both clinical patients and persons, particularly infants suffering from inapparent infections are infectious; both may act as carriers of the virus. This virus may be harbored in the throat for a relatively brief period of several days whereas in the alimentary tract, it generally remains several weeks or more. The infantile carrier 6 to 18 months of age is a particularly dangerous carrier (Gard 1960), owing to the bowel habits of young infants, to the unsuspected nature of the illness, and to the intimate contact between mother and child. Healthy carriers are by far the most numerous and uncontrolled because their symptom-free infection escapes detection by clinicians and health officers alike. Theoretically, then, such cases can act as a huge human reservoir for the spread of the disease and perhaps for the maintenance of the virus in a community during interepidemic periods.

When only frank cases are counted during a poliomyelitis epidemic, it would appear that the disease has a low index of contagion, and for years this was taken for granted. But, if the mild cases and the inapparent infections are included, then poliomyelitis attack rates reveal it to be a highly contagious disease, giving a different impression from that arrived at by counting the paralytic cases alone. This was the impression that Wickman (1905) had gained at the beginning of the century, although he had only scant knowledge of the ratio of abortive to frank cases; Paul, Salinger, and Trask gave this ratio special emphasis in 1931 (1932, 1933).

PATHOGENESIS: PORTALS OF ENTRY

Shortly after the discovery of the virus by Landsteiner and Popper in 1908, Kling *et al.* (1912) in Sweden set out to isolate poliomyelitis virus from the throat and from the feces of clinical cases and thus laid the groundwork for many further clinical and virological investigations of the epidemiology of poliomyelitis. The accumulated evidence indicates that the mouth is the usual portal of entry. Viremia occurs soon after exposure, and the oropharynx and the intestinal tract are sites for the primary implantation of the virus, which apparently localizes largely in lymphoid tissue. The intranasal portal of entry has much less support. The cutaneous route of infection cannot be disregarded. At least with some strains of the virus, infection can be readily induced experimentally by this route in various species of monkey. It has also been demonstrated in man.

In any event it is clear that close human association (contact) is all important (Paffenbarger *et al.* 1954). Susceptibles exposed to an infected person within households acquire high infection rates. This applies to children and even to young adults. Infants under two years (presumably because of their unsanitary habits) are considered the most successful disseminators. Whether polioviruses travel primarily from the oropharynx of one person to another, or whether the fecal-oropharyngeal circuit is the major one has not yet been firmly established. It probably differs under different circumstances. Epidemiologic evidence indicates that a case is most infectious during the early stages of infection, sometime before the onset of second phase symptoms of the clinical disease. This dating of the onset of the disease to second phase symptoms was originally estimated as the incubation period of poliomyelitis—about 10 days. But the shorter period corresponding to the onset of first phase symptoms (when they are present) from the date of exposure, is probably more accurate (Horstmann and Paul 1947). This period lasts 2 to 4 days and shortly after it the virus can be demonstrated in the blood stream and the throat. This might suggest that the pharyngeal-oropharyngeal route is the more important route of dissemination.

There are also a number of facts that support the view that poliomyelitis is an enteric infection spread primarily by contaminated excreta. First, virus dissemination is facilitated by a poor sanitary environment, a feature that is not paralleled in at least some infections spread by the respiratory route. Second, evidence exists that the period of infectiousness parallels closely the period of maximum fecal excretion of virus. Finally, studies with oral vaccine indicate that spread from vaccinees to contacts can occur even though no demonstrable virus is present in the throat (Fox *et al.* 1961), and in some instances when throat infection has been completely bypassed by feeding virus in capsules (Koprowski *et al.* 1956, Horstmann'*et al.* 1959).

At present there is mounting evidence that both pharyngeal and fecal mechanisms of spread operate. In populations living in poor sanitary conditions where much fecal contamination exists, the fecal-oropharyngeal route is quite possibly of greater importance and accounts for the high rate of poliovirus circulation among young children.

DISTRIBUTION OF VIRUS IN THE BODY AND PORTALS OF EXIT

Early in the incubation period in man the virus has been recovered from the blood stream. How frequently viremia occurs in the natural disease is not known. It is there within a very few days, lasting sometimes two to five days after the ingestion of monovalent Type II (Sabin) oral vaccine. Viremia has been noted rarely, if at all, with the other two types of Sabin attenuated strains (Makay *et al.* 1963, Horstmann *et al.* 1964).

Those individuals who lack antibodies (triple negatives) circulate the virus in the blood stream more commonly than those who are only homotypic negatives. The extent to which this demonstrable viremia indicates the route along which the virus travels from the primary site of implantation through the blood and/or through tissues to reach the blood-brain barrier and pass into the central nervous system (CNS) has not been settled. Although the virus may be widespread in the body early in the clinical disease, it has certain sites of predilection, such as the pharynx, intestine, and CNS, where it survives for varying periods of time. Only in the CNS does it produce serious lesions.

The virus can be demonstrated in the oropharynx for about a week to ten days after onset. In the intestinal tract the virus remains longer (from one to six weeks or even more), and as many as one million infectious doses for the monkey have been detected in a gram of feces. Again it should be emphasized here that this acute and convalescent carrier state can often be initiated by an attack so mild as to go unnoticed. Just what the virus of poliomyelitis is doing in the oropharynx or the intestinal tract and how it is maintained are questions not yet answered. Possibly it is growing in fairly superficial local cells and being eliminated into the oropharynx or into the lumen of the gut. Epidemiologically speaking, it would seem that these are "dangerous places" for a highly infectious virus to be. Although poliovirus may continue to be excreted from the intestinal tract for as long as seventeen weeks from onset, long-term human carriers who excrete virus for years—comparable to persistent carriers in typhoid fever—have not been discovered.

EXTRAHUMAN SOURCES OF POLIOVIRUS

Important as the direct contact explanation for the spread of poliomyelitis is, it may not be the whole answer. In any event it does seem that man can contaminate not only his fellow associates but his immediate environment, and it is possible that on occassion an analogy can be drawn between poliomyelitis and the bacterial diseases of salmonellosis. Poliovirus has been found not only in human feces but, under natural circumstances, in urban sewage and in fecal material collected in open privies (Paul, Trask, and Gard 1940). The presence of poliomyelitis virus in sewage at certain periods of the year does not mean that sewage is the usual avenue of infection. It is merely evidence that the community is contaminated. Tubercle bacilli can, for instance, be found with great frequency in urban sewage; yet one does not regard sewage as the source of tuberculosis in urban communities. Seldom, if ever, has there been laboratory evidence to incriminate the water supply of a community as a source of local poliomyelitis infections. In only a few outbreaks have there been reasons to believe that milk was the source of the infection, but this also has lacked laboratory confirmation.

A variety of arthropods, from time to time, have been suspected of spreading poliomyelitis, largely because of the seasonal incidence. Many varieties of insects have been tested for the presence of virus. Such tests have yielded no positive results except in the case of flies and cockroaches (Gear 1952). It is now clear that various species of flies may carry the virus on their surfaces or within their bodies (Paul *et al.* 1941, Ward Melnick, and Horstmann 1945, Melnick and Penner 1952). Particularly does this apply to the fecal-feeding species. It is clear, also, that naturally infected flies can contaminate food with poliovirus. There is no reason to regard insects as an essential or a dominant element in the spread of this disease, however. In some epidemics that have occurred in the Arctic during the winter, flies could have played no part. On the other hand, in certain areas where sanitary conditions are substandard and flies are exceedingly common, such as in cities or villages in Egypt or South Africa, the role these insects may play as mechanical vectors in spreading the virus of poliomyelitis could be appreciable. The word "mechanical" is used here although there is evidence that poliovirus multiplies slightly in flies. Although flies that have been infected under artificial conditions harbor polioviruses only for about 15 days, cockroaches, on the other hand, have been demonstrated to harbor the virus for 51 days (Davé and Wallis 1965*a, b*).

Polioviruses can contaminate the local environment widely, but no large extrahuman reservoir of virus is recognized as existing apart from the immediate environment of infected people—usually children. None the less, environmental factors do play a part in the spread of this disease. This is primarily manifested by the fact that infection and immunity are so uniformly acquired by infants in areas and communities where infant mortality is high and where poor sanitation and much fecal pollution of the environment exists.

GENERAL CONSIDERATION

Poliomyelitis is apparently one of those diseases that, like measles, is wont to spread into a susceptible population, especially the younger age groups, when the opportunity arises. Today there are few communities, no matter how small or remote, that can hope to escape paralytic cases of the disease for long unless vigorous vaccination programs are pursued. Particularly in communities where the interepidemic period is long does the risk of a potentially severe epidemic increase annually, as a population composed of unvaccinated infants, children, and even young adults is built up. This susceptible population, therefore, is a kind of growing vacuum in which the virus may surge when the opportunity presents itself. Few more graphic examples of this are available than that of the poliomyelitis epidemic among Canadian Eskimos in 1948–49, which has been described by Peart (1949). The disease was then introduced into settlements along the west side of Hudson Bay and spread rapidly northward, reaching the remote settlement of Chesterfield Inlet where almost 60 per cent of the entire population was infected with paralytic disease. The virus attacked all age groups, the lowest clinical attack rate being in the infants! This fact reminds us that, as in measles, the age distribution of cases of poliomyelitis within a community or population can also be taken as an indication of the pre-epidemic immunity of that population, which must have been exceedingly low in these Eskimos.

Today, however, measurements besides those of age-specific rates can actually be made in advance of an epidemic; these may enable the epidemiologist to determine the immune status of a given population from time to time. This matter has been discussed at some length in the chapter on serological epidemiology (see Fig. 21).

In the ten-year period since the introduction of the Salk-type vaccine, the prevalence of the clinical disease has already been enormously reduced in countries that have used vaccines extensively (see Fig. 29). The age-distribution of cases has also been altered. With the Sabin vaccine cases have been further reduced.

Conclusion

Epidemiological thinking about poliomyelitis has undergone a complete revision—a revision that began well before the introduction of the Salk- and Sabin-type vaccines. Originally regarded in the nineteenth century as a disease limited to infants, it is now known to affect all age groups. From being considered mildly contagious or infectious, it is now regarded as highly infectious. From being considered an infection in which the outcome usually included acute paralysis, it is now known that only one person in a hundred or more becomes paralyzed. A disease that was for a time considered a respiratory infection, is now regarded as one of the alimentary tract.

Poliomyelitis behaves differently in different environments. This has been brought out in studies of urban areas where sanitary arrangements are adequate as opposed to areas where they are deficient. In communities where sanitation is primitive and living conditions are crowded and poor, facilities for the spread of such a virus are better than elsewhere. Consequently, infants have the opportunity of coming into contact with all three types of poliovirus early in life, and few of them reach the age of three or four without having been infected with at least one strain, although clinically the infection is largely inapparent. Therefore, immunity is acquired early and silently in such areas, and no large group of susceptibles is built up among children or young adults; the disease continually smolders, and epidemics of poliomyelitis among natives are not likely to occur. In countries where the sanitary arrangements are no longer primitive, the risk of contact with the virus at an early age is diminished. A large percentage of the juvenile population may often reach the age of six, eight, or ten without having acquired any infection or any immunity; consequently such populations are often ripe for epidemics. In none of these populations has the need for vaccination of the juvenile population from at least 6 months to 12 years old been reduced. Profound alterations have been wrought in the epidemiologic picture by the use of vaccines, and no doubt more will come to pass in the near future.

BIBLIOGRAPHY

BADHAM, J. 1836. Paralysis in childhood. Four remarkable cases of suddenly induced paralysis in the extremities. *Lond. Med. Gaz.* **17**:215.

BELL, C. 1836. *The nervous system of the human body as explained in a series of papers.* 3d ed. London: Royal Society of London.

COLMER, G. 1843. Paralysis in teething children. *Am. J. Med. Sci.* **5**:248.

CORDIER, S. 1888. Relation d'une épidémie de paralysie atrophique de l'enfance. *Mem. Comptes rendus Soc. Sci. Med. Lyon.* **27**:289.

DAVÉ, K. H. and WALLIS, R. C. 1965a. Survival of Type 1 and Type 3 polio vaccine viruses in blowflies (*Phaenicia sericata*) at 40° C. *Proc. Soc. Exp. Biol. Med.* **11**:121–24.

———. 1965b. Preliminary communication on the survival, the sites harboring virus and genetic stability of poliovirus in cockroaches. *Ibid.* **119**:124–26.

ENDERS, J. F., WELLER, T. H., and ROBBINS, F. C. 1949. Cultivation of the Lansing strain of poliomyelitis virus in cultures of various human embryonic tissues. *Science* **109**:85–87.

FOX, J. P., GELFAND, H. M., BLATT, P. N., LEBLANC, D. R., and CONWELL, D. P. 1955. Immunizing patterns with poliomyelitis viruses and sero-immune patterns in southern Louisiana. *Ann. N.Y. Acad. Sci.* **61**:968.

FOX, J. P., GELFAND, H. M., LEBLANC, D. R., POTASH, L., CLEMMER, D. I., and LAPENTA, D. 1961. The spread of vaccine strains of poliovirus in the household and in the community in southern Louisiana. In *Poliomyelitis: papers and discussions presented at Fifth International Polio Conference*, p. 368. Philadelphia: J. B. Lippincott Co.

GARD, S. 1960. Field and laboratory experiences with CHAT strain of Type I poliovirus. In *Second International Conference on live poliovirus vaccines*, p. 187. Washington, D.C.: Pan American Sanitary Bureau.

GEAR, J. H. S. 1952. The extrahuman sources of poliomyelitis. In

Papers and discussions presented at the Second International Poliomyelitis Conference, Copenhagen, 1951. Philadelphia: J. B. Lippincott Co.

————. 1955. Poliomyelitis in the underdeveloped areas of the world. In *Poliomyelitis.* W.H.O. Monograph Series, No. 26., p. 31. Geneva.

HEINE, J. 1840. *Beobachtungen über Lähmungszustände der unteren Extremitäten und deren Behandlung.* Stuttgart: Köhler.

HILLMAN, C. C. 1936. Poliomyelitis in the Philippine Islands. *Military Surg.* **79**:48.

HORSTMANN, D. M., NIEDERMAN, J. C., and PAUL, J. R. 1959. Attenuated Type I poliovirus vaccine. Its capacity to infect and to spread from "vaccinees" within an institutional population. *J.A.M.A.* **170**:1–3.

HORSTMANN, D. M., OPTON, E. M., KLEMPERER, R., LLADO, B., and VIGNEC, A. J. 1964. Viremia in infants vaccinated with oral poliovirus vaccine (Sabin). *Am. J. Hyg.* **79**:47–63.

HORSTMANN, D. M. and PAUL, J. R. 1947. The incubation period in human poliomyelitis virus and its implications. *J.A.M.A.* **135**:11–14.

KLING, C., PETTERSSON, A., and WERNSTEDT, W. 1912. The presence of the microbe of infantile paralysis in human beings. *Comm. Inst. Med. Stockholm* **3**:5.

KOPROWSKI, H. 1961. Influence of age on susceptibility to infection with live attenuated poliovirus. In *Poliomyelitis, papers and discussions presented at the Fifth International Poliomyelitis Conference,* p. 290. Philadelphia: J. B. Lippincott. Co.

LANDSTEINER, K. and POPPER, E. 1908. Mikroscopische Präparate von einem Menschlichen und zwei Affenrückenmarken. *Wien. klin. Wochnschr.* **21**:1830.

MEDIN, O. 1891. *Über eine Epidemie von spinaler Kinderlähmung Verhandl. X. Internat. med. Kongr.* **2**:37.

MELNICK, J. L. and LEDINKO, N. 1953. Development of neutralizing antibodies against the 3 types of poliomyelitis virus during an epidemic period: The ratio of inapparent infection to clinical poliomyelitis. *Am. J. Hyg.* **58**:207.

OLIN, G. 1952. The epidemiological pattern of poliomyelitis in Sweden from 1905 to 1950. In *Papers and discussions presented at the Second International Poliomyelitis Conference, Copenhagen, 1951.* Philadelphia: J. B. Lippincott Co.

OLIN, G. and WESSLEN, T. 1957. Seroimmune patterns for poliomyelitis in Sweden. *Arch. Ges. Virusforsch.* **1**:13.

PAFFENBERGER, R. S., WILSON, V. O., BODIAN, D., and WATT, J. 1954. The spread of poliomyelitis. An analysis of contact during epidemic periods. *Am. J. Hyg.* **60**:63.

PAUL, J. R. 1949. Poliomyelitis attack rates in American troops, 1940–1948. *Am. J. Hyg.* **50**:57.

———. 1955. *Epidemiology of poliomyelitis.* Monograph Series No. 26. Geneva: World Health Organization.

———. 1958. Endemic and epidemic trends of poliomyelitis in Central and South America. Bull. *World Health Organ.* **19**:747.

PAUL, J. R., MELNICK, J. L., BARNETT, V. H., and GOLDBLUM, N. 1952. A survey of neutralizing antibodies to poliomyelitis virus in Cairo, Egypt. *Am. J. Hyg.* **55**:402.

PAUL, J. R., MELNICK, J. L., and RIORDAN, J. T. 1952. Comparative neutralizing antibody patterns to Lansing (Type 2) poliomyelitis virus in different populations. *Am. J. Hyg.* **56**:232.

PAUL, J. R. and RIORDAN, J. T. 1950. Observations on serological epidemiology: Antibodies to the Lansing strain of poliomyelitis virus in sera from Alaskan Eskimos. *Am. J. Hyg.* **52**:202.

PAUL, J. R., SALINGER, R., and TRASK, J. D. 1932. "Abortive" poliomyelitis. *J.A.M.A.* **9**:2262.

———. 1933. Studies on the epidemiology of poliomyelitis. II. Incidence of abortive types of poliomyelitis. *Am. J. Hyg.* **19**:587–600.

PAYNE, A. M-M. 1955. Poliomyelitis as a world problem. In *Poliomyelitis. Papers and discussions presented at the Third International Poliomyelitis Conference,* p. 393. Philadelphia: J. B. Lippincott Co.

PEART, A. F. W. 1949. An outbreak of poliomyelitis in Canadian Eskimos in wintertime; epidemiological features. *Can. J. Public Health* **40**:405–17.

RIORDAN, J. T., PAUL, J. R., YOSHIOKA, I., and HORSTMANN, D. M. 1961. The detection of poliovirus and other enteric viruses in flies. Results of tests carried out during an oral poliovirus vaccine trial. *Am. J. Hyg.* **74**:123–36.

SABIN, A. B. 1962. Oral poliovirus vaccine. Recent results and recommendations for optimum use. *Roy. Soc. Health J.* **82**:51–59.

———. 1963. Poliomyelitis in the tropics. Increasing incidence and prospects for control. *Trop. Geograph. Med.* **15**:38.

SALK, J. E. 1955. A concept of the mechanism of immunity for preventing paralysis in poliomyelitis. *Ann. N.Y. Acad. Sci.* **61**:1023.

TRASK, J. D., PAUL, J. R., and MELNICK, J. L. 1943. Detection of poliomyelitis virus in flies collected during epidemics of poliomyelitis: Methods, results, and types of flies involved. *J. Exp. Med.* **77**:531.

WARD, R., MELNICK, J. L., and HORSTMANN, D. M. 1945. Poliomyelitis virus in fly-contaminated food collected at an epidemic. *Science* **101**:491–93.

CHAPTER XVII

Infectious and Serum Hepatitis

This disease (or group of diseases) has been chosen as an example of a viral infection to which the medical and surgical profession of two hemispheres has devoted special attention during the past twenty years. This marks the short period during which revised concepts have arisen regarding hepatitis—its nomenclature, pathogenesis, and epidemiology.

Presumably, infectious hepatitis is an example of the enteric group of infectious diseases. Serum hepatitis (the other member of the family which has been split off arbitrarily) has many features that do not belong in the enteric category at all and, epidemiologically speaking, that are almost unique. It is one of the "man-made diseases," and its increasing prevalence reflects the increasing use of transfusions, blood products, and inoculations of all kinds in the practice of modern medicine. Many of its epidemiological features are still obscure, and it may be too soon to attempt to document them. But at the risk of being premature and inadequate, some of the known facts will be listed.

HISTORY

Viral hepatitis is certainly an old disease, long recognized in civilian and military medical history under a variety of different names. Its current prominence stems not only from its baffling etiology, its frequency and occasional seriousness but from the development of new concepts of pathogenesis and from the significance attached to its current name—in other words, its nosography. As long as most cases of viral hepatitis masqueraded under the name of "acute catarrhal jaundice" (regarded as a mild though common illness) and another "acute yellow atrophy of the liver" (regarded as a rare but serious disease), this

196

disease occupied a back seat. That was prior to 1940. Now both diseases are regarded as the same, namely a virus disease that in adults can have moderately serious implications, and whose name implies contagion. Much of this new concept about its pathogenesis came with the realization that this type of jaundice was not due to obstruction of the common bile duct with a mucus plug but instead to a destructive lesion of the liver parenchyma.

Epidemics of jaundice had been recognized for centuries, perhaps most prominently in military medical history; but apart from its infectious nature, the disease had long been poorly defined and poorly described. Prior to the 1880's, infectious hepatitis was often confused with Weil's disease, but subsequently leptospirosis was differentiated by immunologic tests. Among pioneers who assisted in defining infectious hepatitis as a clinical and pathological entity were Quincke (1903), Cockayne (1912), and Eppinger (1922). Blumer (1923) was among the first in the United States to claim that infectious hepatitis probably represented the epidemic form of catarrhal jaundice. Not long after this Rich (1930) drew attention to the universal presence at necropsy of a diffuse hepatitis in cases clinically diagnosed as catarrhal jaundice.

Furthermore, the epidemic potentialities of this disease were brought forcibly to the attention of the medical profession during World War II, when hepatitis became a problem of great magnitude in many armies. In the United States Army, the total number of cases of infectious hepatitis rose to at least 120,000 and, if serum hepatitis cases are added, to about 180,000. This stands in contrast to the mere thirteen lines on the subject of "infectious jaundice," probably cases of leptospirosis, in the history of the Medical Department of the United States Army for World War I.

Modern concepts of the viral etiology of hepatitis and the supposition that two forms of human hepatitis might exist, stem originally from the observations of Flaum *et al.* (1926) in Sweden. They first suggested that patients acquiring hepatitis in a diabetic clinic were infected by contaminated syringes and that the two forms could be distinguished by the length of the incubation periods. Later, Findlay *et al.* (1939) in West Africa and various observers in Brazil described cases of postvaccinal (yellow fever vaccine) hepatitis.

In 1942, Voegt in Germany was the first to report the oral transmission of infectious hepatitis from man to man; he fed the duodenal contents from a patient suffering from this illness to his subjects. Subsequently, others (Havens *et al.* 1944, Neefe *et al.* 1945) found the etiologic agent in the blood and feces and demonstrated that it was capable of passing bacteria-tight filters, and that it could be transmitted serially to human volunteers.

HEPATITIS VIRUSES

Granted that there may be several strains of human infectious hepatitis viruses, perhaps a whole family, the actual causative agent or agents of infectious hepatitis are unknown. The human hepatitis viruses have not yet been seen, in spite of the pictures shown in advertising literature, nor have they yet been definitely isolated or cultured satisfactorily. There are several "candidate viruses," however, but these are still awaiting confirmation. Curiously enough these candidates belong to a multiplicity of different types: Echo, Coxsackie, adenoviruses, herpes simplex, and other unidentified varieties. Some non-human hepatitis viruses have been identified within the past twenty-five years or so, both murine and canine, but these seem to be limited in their host range and have no relation to human varieties.

Our discussion of human hepatitis virus will deal with observations made on infectious agents that have been transmitted to volunteers, who in turn have come down either with infectious or serum hepatitis as a result of the procedure. Using this awkward method a great deal has been learned, and a major division of human hepatitis agents has been established by which infectious hepatitis virus (so-called virus IH, or A virus) has been separated from the serum hepatitis viruses (so-called SH, or B virus). The known properties of these two groups are set forth in Table 5. Both groups are quite resistant to physical and chemical agents, and can withstand being heated at 56° C for thirty minutes, as well as high-level chlorination, and the action of certain other chemicals that ordinarily destroy bacteria.

Some have questioned the wisdom of dividing these two forms of viral hepatitis into separate categories. It can be readily said in

TABLE 5

Comparison of Certain Features of Infectious Hepatitis and Serum Hepatitis and Their Causative Viruses

Clinical and Epidemiologic Features	Infectious Hepatitis	Serum Hepatitis
Incubation period	15 to 40 days	60 to 160 days
Type of onset	Acute	Insidious
Fever—over 38° C (100.4° F)	Common	Uncommon
Seasonal incidence	Autumn-winter	Year round
Age preference	Children and young adults	Any age
	Virus	Virus
Filtrability:		
Seitz EK filter	Passed	Passed
Gradocol membrane with pore size 52 mμ	Not done	Passed
Susceptible host	Man	Man
Virus in feces	Incubation period and acute phase	Not demonstrated
Virus in duodenal contents	Acute phase	Not done
Virus in blood	Incubation period and acute phase	Incubation period and acute phase
Route of infection (experimental)	Oral and parenteral	Parenteral
Duration of carrier state:		
blood	As long as 8 months (one adult)	As long as 5 years (one adult)
feces	As long as 16 months (one child)	Not demonstrated
Immunity:		
homologous	Present	Inconstant
heterologous	None apparent	None apparent
Prophylactic value of gamma globulin	Good	Demonstrated experimentally

defense of such a division, however, that there seems to have been less confusion about this family of diseases since the division became accepted than before.

Infectious Hepatitis:

Clinical Picture and Pathogenesis

A word about the clinical picture of infectious hepatitis and its probable pathologic basis might be helpful. This will of necessity be brief, primarily because so little factual data about the latter is available.

The incubation period averages 20–25 days. The usual clinical course has been arbitrarily divided into preicteric and icteric phases that together may last from three to six weeks. In childhood the disease is very common and often not diagnosed, for the clinical course is shorter and milder; indeed in infants it may escape notice altogether until its presence is felt when nurses or attendants acquire the overt disease. Yet in both adults and children, jaundice may be absent in a sizable percentage of infections. A conservative estimate of the ratio in adults might be 1:1. But among children, Ward and Krugman (1961) have suggested a ratio of nonicteric to icteric as high as 12:1. It could be even higher in infants, a point of fundamental epidemiologic significance. Considering that the majority of patients with hepatitis are already in the relatively late icteric phase by the time the diagnosis is made, most physicians are far more familiar with this aspect of the disease than the aspects of the first phase.

Little is known about the pathogenesis of infectious hepatitis. It is generally assumed that there is an initial viral infection, although the lesions in this preicteric phase, being less evident and certainly less spectacular than those of the icteric phase, have received less attention than they deserve. It has often been asked whether following the preicteric phase some form of autoimmune process which is responsible for the liver damage, might be operative. Indeed certain associated phenomena, such as arthralgia and urticaria strengthen this suggestion. Of possible significance also are the pathologic changes in the icteric phase of hepatitis found in the liver. They are indistinguishable from those found in some patients as manifestations of certain drug reactions.

GEOGRAPHIC DISTRIBUTION

In spite of inadequate information, there is little question that viral hepatitis, perhaps in both forms, is very widespread.[1]

[1] In reporting cases the differentiation between infectious and serum hepatitis is seldom made because the clinical picture of the two is almost identical.

Infectious hepatitis (IH) probably occurs in nearly all inhabited areas of the globe, although there are certain regions with an established record of high endemic prevalence for infectious hepatitis, of which the Far East and the Mediterranean littoral are examples. Military outbreaks are proverbial in these two regions; over the past 150 years these have occurred repeatedly among troops brought into these endemic areas from Europe, Australia, and the North American continent.

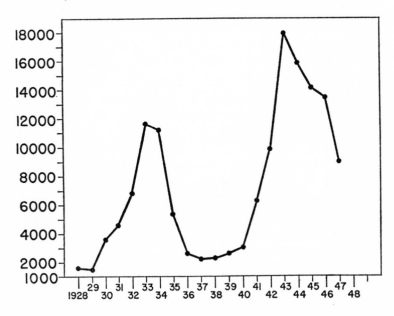

HEPATITIS IN DENMARK 1928–1947
Total Cases

FIG. 31. Cases of hepatitis as recorded in Denmark over a 20-year period (1928–47). (Data from the Danish Ministry of Health, collected by W. P. Havens.)

In Scandinavian countries, long-term information on the incidence of hepatitis has been more complete than elsewhere, and I will turn to them for data on its frequency in that area. This disease has been notifiable in Denmark, for instance, since 1928 (Fig. 31). The experience in Denmark has been in keeping with that of some other countries in temperate climates in which sanitary facilities are standard or above. The incidence has varied greatly with waves of high incidence covering several years, notably the war years, when the country was occupied by German troops. This periodicity of waves of high incidence coming at intervals of nine or ten years and reflecting increases of cases by eight or nine times is not uncommon. How representative of northern Europe this picture may be is not known. In occupied Germany during the years immediately following World War II (1946–51), hepatitis was a constant scourge to American troops, the incidence reaching at one time the incredibly high rate of 17 per 1,000 (Paul and Gardner 1953). This continued wave of high incidence has generally been ascribed to the damaged plumbing and the associated breakdown in sanitary facilities which beset the devastated cities of that part of Germany in postwar times (1946–52). It is unlikely that the Scandinavian incidence picture or that of northern Europe would be similar to that of a tropical country or one with continued substandard environmental sanitary conditions.

In the United States as a whole, the reporting of cases during the past decade has been irregular and often on a voluntary basis. This situation is now being rectified. In the United States

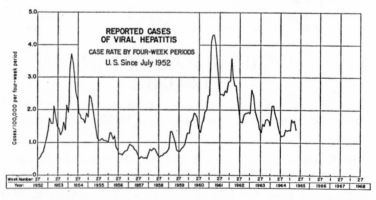

Fig. 32. Incidence rates by four-week periods of cases of viral hepatitis, United States, 1952–65. (Data from Hepatitis Surveillance Reports, U.S. Public Health Service, Atlanta, Ga.)

we face a great variety of climates and living conditions. The chart in Fig. 32 records the over-all experience of at least 13 years, since 1952. Here the peak between the years of high incidence represents about 8 years. This chart shows an almost universal tendency for an annual upswing of cases to begin in late summer. That infectious and/or serum hepatitis is a relatively common disease throughout the nation few would deny.

TRANSMISSION

Most current evidence indicates that infectious hepatitis is usually spread through some form of person-to-person association, although water-borne, food-borne (notably by shellfish) and milk-borne epidemics have been described. Nevertheless, man represents the main source and reservoir of the infection. Otherwise, a nonhuman source of virus has been infected chimpanzees that for the most part have been imported as young and susceptible animals. This discovery has recently received much attention since the observations by Hillis (1961) of eleven cases of hepatitis occurring among personnel working with chimpanzees at an air force base. Following this report a number of small outbreaks of human cases associated with chimpanzees have occurred. Increasing evidence suggests that susceptible chimpanzees may become infected with and may transmit infectious hepatitis virus, although in the past many experimental attempts to infect them have failed, presumably because susceptible animals are difficult to come by. As yet no other extrahuman living host such as an animal, bird, or arthropod has been found in which human hepatitis viruses are known to multiply or survive; the possibility of mechanical transmission by a biting insect has never been eliminated, nor however, has it been adequately investigated. Media, such as water and food, in which these hardy viruses can survive are, of course, well recognized.

There is good evidence to indicate that the intestinal-oral circuit plays a dominant part in the natural person-to-person spread. This is based upon experimental tests with human volunteers, which indicate the frequency with which hepatitis virus (IH) is found in human feces during acute stages of the disease and the ease with which this disease may be produced by feeding such material to man. Although some epidemiologic observations point to a respiratory mode of spread, none of the tests on this has been sufficiently satisfactory (owing to technical or other reasons) for definite conclusions to be drawn from the results. In any event a respiratory type of spread seems unlikely. As with poliomyelitis, personal and close contact with infective people, particularly children, probably accounts for the great majority of orally acquired cases of infectious hepatitis.

The duration of the period of infectivity in the acute case is not known, but the virus is usually excreted in the feces during the active phase of the disease and perhaps for some days afterward. In infants, however, the carrier state may be protracted for months.

Evidence to substantiate that the intestinal-oral circuit is involved is based on the water-borne epidemics of infectious hepatitis just mentioned and the seasonal rises in incidence in summer and early autumn (see Fig. 33). Unlike a variety of enteric infections, its season often extends throughout the winter. This extension into the winter months has been invoked many times to indicate that the respiratory tract plays an active part in the transmission of infectious hepatitis. This may possibly be true, although the epidemic season often begins, in areas of poor sanitation or where sanitary rules break down, during the season when enteric diseases are most apt to appear and once started may well run a prolonged course.

Often outbreaks of hepatitis are preceded by a wave of gastroenteric illness, presumably of bacterial origin. This experience often occurred in North Africa during World War II. Military records also state that hepatitis incidence is highest when and where the sanitation of camps is poor.

Civilian evidence further testifies to the frequency with which visitors acquire hepatitis in tropical or semitropical areas when they come in contact with poor sanitary conditions. In institutions for mentally deficient individuals, hepatitis rates have been higher in those buildings housing individuals with the lowest mental capacities and, therefore, those in which sanitary standards are maintained with the greatest difficulty.

But it should again be emphasized that, since viral hepatitis is easily spread by intimate association among people, epidemics of this disease may and do occur frequently where sanitary facilities are far from substandard, in well-run institutions, homes, and

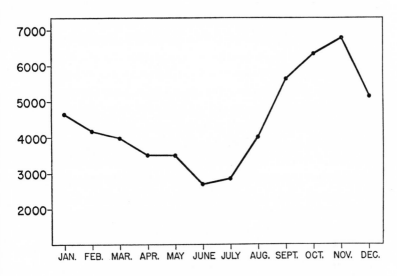

HEPATITIS IN SWEDEN 1931—1947
Total Cases

Fig. 33. Seasonal pattern of hepatitis in Sweden over a 17-year period, 1931–47. (Data collected by W. P. Havens.)

apartment buildings. Outbreaks certainly occur in the best of regulated families. Often involved are housing projects where the proportion of children in the population is above average. Within some of these communities, it may well be that a large unsuspected source of virus maintains itself periodically in the form of inapparent, infantile, or juvenile subclinical cases. Under these circumstances, it is small wonder that the disease spreads readily to the susceptibles in the exposed population group.

Man continues to be the most generally recognized source of infectious hepatitis virus; and it has long been known that the virus can be recovered from blood and feces in the active stages of icteric cases (Havens 1946a) as well as from nonicteric cases, where it may be transmitted to volunteers by feeding or by parenteral inoculation. Krugman and Giles * have recently described the transmission of hepatitis by feeding urine obtained from patients in the preicteric phase of disease, but how important viruria is in the dissemination of the disease is unknown.

Krugman *et al.* (1959) have shown that virus may be present in the latter part of the incubation period, two or three weeks prior to the appearance of jaundice. How long virus remains in blood and feces after the onset of the disease is problematic; it has generally been absent when tested 1 to 13 months after onset. Nevertheless Murray *et al.* (1955) have made demonstrations of viremia in an adult patient 8 months after onset and Capps *et al.* (1952) have demonstrated it in infants 5 and 14 months old. A certain percentage of recipients of transfusions have acquired hepatitis after a short incubation period, and this suggests that the carrier state of IH virus in the blood may exist more frequently than has been previously suspected.

TYPES OF EPIDEMICS

1. Water-borne. There are now many good examples of the explosive water-borne epidemic, notably two that occurred in summer camps (Neefe and Stokes 1945, Tucker and Farrel 1954). In the one reported by Tucker and Farrel, which occurred at a church camp in Tennessee, there were two separate waves of infections. It was suggested that both infections, acute gastroenteritis and infectious hepatitis, were related to the same source and the differences in the lengths of the respective incubation periods (a few days for gastroenteritis and about three weeks for infectious hepatitis) gave rise to two sequential waves of illness.

* S. Krugman and J. P. Giles, 1963, unpublished material.

Another recent example of a huge water-borne urban epidemic of infectious hepatitis was reported in 1956 in Delhi, India. Cases are said to have numbered around 30,000. Melnick (1956) reported that the Delhi water supply became contaminated with sewage through an accidental shift in the course of a neighboring river. An alert sanitary engineer immediately increased the chlorine concentration in the city water supply, and no noticeable increase in the rate of cases of acute gastroenteritis was recorded. A month later the hepatitis epidemic began, however. The increased concentration of chlorine had apparently been effective in destroying bacterial pathogenic agents but was ineffective with the hepatitis virus.

2. *Food-handlers and the spread of hepatitis.* It is more than likely that food-handlers, during the various infectious stages of inapparent or clinical hepatitis, play an important part in the spread of IH virus. This has also been documented in military experience. During World War II one bit of oft-quoted evidence was the higher rate of infectious hepatitis among officers as opposed to enlisted men, a differential that was more prominent among British troops in Italy, for instance, than among American troops. As a group, the officers may well have been more susceptible, but another explanation of the high rates among them was that they ate in a mess where natives acted as waiters (food-handlers); the enlisted men had their own cooks and served themselves.

Salads and milk have often been readily contaminated by an infected food-handler. The outbreaks attributed to shellfish in this country have nearly always been traced to the ingestion of raw oysters or clams, which have been harvested (illegally, it may be unnecessary to add) in polluted waters. In tracing such outbreaks a useful measure has been to analyze the age distribution of cases. Unlike the age distribution in many epidemics of hepatitis, cases in shellfish epidemics have occurred almost entirely in adults. As a rule children do not care for raw shellfish.

3. *Institutional outbreaks.* These are common in orphan asylums, boarding schools, and notoriously so in mental institutions.

In some large mental institutions with a population of 2,000 or more, hepatitis and salmonellosis may become endemic, and over the course of several years cases may continue to appear in large or small numbers each month, both in inmates and attendants. This situation has been ascribed to the bowel habits of mentally deficient inmates, be they children or adults, and to the great difficulties of maintaining adequate standards of environmental sanitation even in the best-run institutions (Ward and Krugman 1958).

4. Family epidemics. These are so common and well known that they hardly deserve mention. The usual story, in a family of four or five members, is that one child contracts a mild case of "jaundice" first, and not much is made of it. About a month later another child and/or perhaps a parent becomes jaundiced. Usually much more attention is paid to the adult case, although to the epidemiologist all cases would be of equal importance. The long interval between cases offers an opportunity to apply the use of gamma globulin as a prophylactic measure in such situations.

AGE DISTRIBUTION

Under most circumstances, and in areas where hepatitis is common, the disease is essentially one of childhood (Horstmann, Havens, and Deutsch 1947). Indeed, children are said to account for 65 per cent of the cases, with the bulk of them occurring between the ages of five and eighteen, as Fig. 34 graphically demonstrates. It is obvious that this may vary considerably under different environmental conditions or at different times in the same place. The concentration of the disease in juveniles has been responsible for many misconceptions about local incidence, because juvenile cases are apt to be so mild that they escape recognition, and the adult population, being immune, yields relatively few cases. Often a community is completely unaware of the high local incidence of infections due to hepatitis virus or its potential danger to visitors. This is in keeping with the epidemiologic behavior of other infections that confer immunity, such as poliomyelitis, whose ready and inapparent spread among

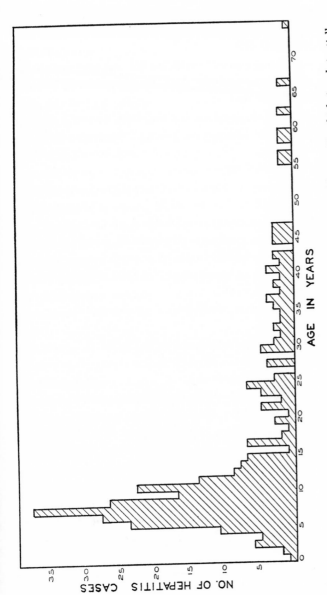

FIG. 34. The age incidence of epidemic hepatitis in Germany prior to World War II, which is substantially the same as it is in the United States today in the usual urban epidemic of viral hepatitis. (Data from two outbreaks occurring in Hamburg and Wilhelmsberg, described by Holm in 1939 and quoted by von Bormann, 1940. *Ergeb. inn. Med. Kinderheilk.* **58**:201.)

local infants is facilitated by inadequate sanitation. Within such areas, hepatitis infection and immunity is acquired so early in life that mild diarrhea may be the only symptom. Superficially, therefore, the disease often seems to be conspicuous by its absence, but it makes its presence known when susceptible visitors enter the endemic area.

This mildness of infantile and childhood hepatitis has not received the emphasis it deserves, particularly since there is no evidence that such mild cases are any the less infectious; indeed, because the duration of the intestinal carrier state in infants is so prolonged, they may be more infectious. The observations of Capps and Stokes (1952, also see Stokes *et al.* 1954), who have described outbreaks in institutions for the care of infants, showed that the clinical disease came to the surface when susceptible adults, such as nurses, were brought in intimate contact with the infectious but apparently healthy babies. In this sense these long-term infant carriers can actually serve as a reservoir of infection, as dangerous to their own small cosmos as was the Broad Street pump.

Although incidence rates are apt to be lower in adults than children, the severity of the clinical disease increases sharply in adult groups, with a rising case fatality rate in age groups over thirty. Correspondingly, it is likely that the ratio of inapparent to overt cases shifts with advancing age, the overt cases becoming relatively more common.

SEX DISTRIBUTION

From the scanty data available for analysis, cases of viral hepatitis seem to be evenly distributed between the two sexes. In some series of cases, however, female parents of childbearing age may acquire hepatitis at a slightly higher rate than males of a comparable age. It is presumed that, as with poliomyelitis, the mother's closer intimacy with the infectious children, particularly those under 18 months, may be responsible for this effect.

IMMUNITY AND IMMUNE REACTIONS

It is ordinarily believed that homologous immunity is conferred by one attack of IH and perhaps also by SH, but not heterologous immunity between IH and SH. The age distribution of IH in most urban populations substantiates this, inasmuch as, far more cases are recorded among juveniles than adults (Fig. 34). Furthermore the susceptibility of military personnel to acquire IH who have recovered from a post-vaccinal attack of SH is often quoted. The demonstration that human gamma globulin is such an effective preventive measure for IH when administered in the incubation period suggests the presence of a humoral substance in the blood of immune persons. True this homologous immunity may not be completely solid in some persons recovered from IH infections, particularly in areas where there is heavy exposure. Thus a reinfection rate of about four per cent has been recorded in a state institution for mentally deficient children. Of course, this could conceivably be due to a multiplicity of IH strains (Ward *et al.* 1960) or even of a mixture of IH and SH strains.

Satisfactory studies of IH immunity suffer because of a lack of immunological tests. A number of nonspecific serologic reactions have been reviewed by Havens (1954, 1963). Notable among them are agglutinins for erythrocytes of various vertebrate species including day old chicks, monkeys, and man, but their limited value makes it hardly worth recording them here.

SERUM HEPATITIS

Virus A of infectious hepatitis (IH) and virus B of serum hepatitis (SH), of which there may be several varieties, may well be variants of a stem organism. Each main group of these viruses (IH and SH) has characteristic properties which give rise to certain different epidemiological situations (see Table 5).

Our knowledge of the epidemiology of serum hepatitis has suffered from the fact that the clinical disease caused by SH virus (or viruses) is almost indistinguishable from infectious hepatitis, so that the two are nearly always reported as one and the same disease. Most notable among the readily detected differences is that the SH incubation period is much longer than that of IH.

Although the recorded incidence rates of serum hepatitis are far below those of infectious hepatitis, the rate of SH is probably actually increasing in this country. As was mentioned at the beginning of this chapter, the mounting use of blood transfusions, of blood products, and of a variety of inoculations or parenteral therapy all offer a growing opportunity for the inadvertent transmission of serum hepatitis virus. Infectious hepatitis may, of course, also be transmitted parenterally, but because its viremic stage is usually shorter than that of serum hepatitis, the likelihood of artificial transmission of infectious hepatitis is less. Thus the best-known vector of serum hepatitis is the syringe, although it is safe to say that the virus of SH did not originate in a syringe, nor does it multiply therein. The strong resistance of hepatitis viruses to various physical and chemical agents, the infectivity of very small doses of the etiologic agent, and the frequency and prolonged duration of the carrier (viremic) state in serum hepatitis in man are important determining factors in facilitating its transmission, and as such they condition its epidemiology.

Observations on the period of infectivity designed to determine when SH viremia is present have indicated a far longer period than in IH hepatitis. SH viremia has been noted in the incubation period 87 days before the onset of jaundice (Paul *et al.* 1945). The studies of Stokes *et al.* (1954) recorded several blood donors who had carried SH virus in their blood for periods ranging from one to five years. Some of these donors showed low-grade chronic liver dysfunction, but it is very difficult to detect with certainty or to determine the frequency of such cases in the general population by the use of liver function tests (see also Neefe *et al.* 1954). A subsequent observation by Murray *et al.* (1955) revealed viremia in one patient after recovery, when all tests for hepatic function were normal. At any rate, evidence suggests that the carrier (viremic) state, either transient or prolonged, may exist more than had been suspected previously.

HISTORY

Although serum hepatitis has long been in existence, its earliest recorded examples are those epidemics following vaccination for smallpox in Germany in the 1880's (Lürman 1885). I have already referred to the cogent observation by Flaum *et al.* (1926) in a diabetic clinic in Sweden. There were some other records of small outbreaks, but little was heard of this kind of jaundice until the 1930's and 1940's when thousands of cases resulted from injections of yellow fever vaccine containing contaminated human serum (Findlay *et al.* 1939, Fox *et al.* 1942, and Sawyer *et al.* 1944). Subsequently this risk of a contaminated vaccine has been eliminated.

MODES OF TRANSMISSION

The potential risk of serum hepatitis occurs in a multiplicity of unsuspected ways: by the improper sterilization of syringes, needles, or instruments employed in giving medications or withdrawing blood; in transfusions of whole blood or plasma (particularly pooled plasma) or in the administration of fibrinogen or thrombin; various dental procedures, and even tattooing has been held responsible. It is not our intent to imply that serum hepatitis must only, or always, be transmitted artificially through a needle or instrument. It is conceivable that certain forms of intimate association between people can transmit SH virus (or strains intermediate between IH and SH), although actual examples of this mode of transmission are few.

DISTRIBUTION AND PREVALENCE OF SERUM HEPATITIS

Serum hepatitis undoubtedly may occur wherever human blood or its products are given parenterally, or accidentally, provided there are local carriers of SH virus, particularly long-term carriers, within the community. Little is known about the world distribution of such carriers, but serum hepatitis has been described in such widely separated areas as the United States, Russia, England, Sweden, and the Middle East. Since transfusions, inoculations, and so forth usually continue at much the same rate throughout the year, serum hepatitis shows little of the seasonal fluctuation so prominent in the monthly incidence rates of infectious hepatitis (Fig. 33). Consequently, the nonseasonal behavior of serum hepatitis has sometimes been used as a measure of differentiating cases of SH from IH (Paul and Gardner 1950).

OUTBREAKS OF SERUM HEPATITIS

These commonly result from the more or less simultaneous inoculation of numbers of people with blood or blood products that have been inadvertently contaminated with SH virus. An outstanding example of this occurred among U.S. troops in World War II, following inoculations with contaminated yellow fever vaccine, an accident that yielded more than 60,000 cases (Sawyer *et al.* 1944, Parr 1945). A long, but variable, interval between the time of infection and the development of the disease is a characteristic feature of serum hepatitis, which has an incubation period considerably longer than that of infectious hepatitis. It has often made the task of tracing the source of the infection very difficult. In the camp epidemic referred to and depicted in Fig. 13, individual differences in the incubation period ranged from 60 to 140 days in 1,004 men who all contracted serum hepatitis after receiving simultaneously the same dose of SH virus. The case incidence curve might have suggested an illness transmitted sequentially from person to person rather than a common-source epidemic, had not the source of the outbreak been known.

Of particular importance during the past few years has been the recognition of outbreaks in clinics where incompletely sterilized instruments were used and where the chances of contamination by carriers of virus were frequent. Diabetic clinics, hematology clinics, and dental clinics (Folley and Gutheim 1956) are examples. Characteristically, these cases appeared in a straggling manner throughout the year, apparently dependent in part on the number of carriers and the degree of cleansing and sterilization of the equipment. The pattern of such outbreaks may be influenced by the fact that IH virus may be transmitted parenterally along with SH virus. Wewalka (1953) has described two interesting groups of cases in which this occurred in a clinic for antiluetic therapy; he observed both short and long incubation-period hepatitis in the same patient.

The potential magnitude of risk of SH hepatitis is attested to by the 21.9 per cent incidence (which is an extreme) of certain groups of post-transfusion cases in soldiers, that is, in those receiving transfusions of blood and plasma; and the 3.6 per cent incidence of other groups receiving whole blood in the Korean War. Among civilians, the post-transfusion incidence depends on many variables but has usually not reached anything like the military proportions (Stokes 1962).

AGE DISTRIBUTION

All age groups are susceptible to serum hepatitis. The disease has been said to be milder in children, although serious outbreaks among infants, with high mortality, have been recorded. Since it is impossible to measure the immune response following infection with SH virus, it is not known whether this general susceptibility of all ages is due to: (*a*) the route of inoculation, (*b*) heavy dosage, (*c*) limited previous exposure of the population to SH virus, (*d*) the failure to develop adequate immunity following exposure, or (*e*) the existence of multiple strains of virus that are immunologically unrelated. The severity of disease and the mortality in previously healthy young adults may be similar to those in infectious hepatitis, but more older people acquire serum hepatitis because the disease most often results from "adult procedures." When patients of any age are already debilitated by illness or wounds, the mortality of serum hepatitis increases sharply. The degree of protection gained from the use of gamma globulin in serum hepatitis is not as definite as in IH, but it has been shown to be more or less effective (Myrick *et al.* 1962).

OCCUPATION AND HABITS

There are a few occupational groups, such as physicians and medical technicians, in which the recorded hepatitis attack rates are higher than in the general population (Kuh and Ward 1950, Trumbull and Greiner 1951). Among technical assistants in blood banks, hepatitis has been described as an "occupational disease," and presumably most of this is serum hepatitis. Drug addicts are a small population group in which serum hepatitis (or "syringe hepatitis," as it has been called) is understandably common. Recently, tattooed individuals have been found to be prone to acquire the disease (Smith 1950).

IMMUNITY

Immunity is poorly defined, particularly because of the paucity of knowledge regarding the multiplicity of strains of SH virus. Patients at great risk, such as narcotic addicts, have sustained multiple attacks of hepatitis. On the other hand, there is evidence of homologous immunity since a large percentage of either volunteers or patients who have received contaminated blood or plasma have failed to contract the disease. This suggests an inherent or acquired resistance in the recipients.

In recent studies, Myrick *et al.* (1962) attempted to modify the course of the post-transfusion disease, or eliminate it, by two injections of gamma globulin in amounts of 10 ml., 30 days apart. The studies have yielded adequate statistical data to indicate that almost two thirds of the cases can be prevented by such procedure. At present, however, it would be a highly impractical measure to try to introduce into civilian practice because of the great frequency with which transfusions are employed and the inordinant amounts of gamma globulin that would be required.

CONCLUSION

The *work* of the epidemiologist concerned with the behavior of viral hepatitis would seem to have just begun. One member of these two clinically indistinguishable members of the viral hepatitis family (IH) seems to fall largely into the category of enteric diseases; the other (SH) falls into the category of syringe, or instrument-borne, infections. Information is lacking on the nature of the biologic relationship between these two members of the same family of viruses.

BIBLIOGRAPHY

BLUMER, G. 1923. Infectious jaundice in the United States. *J.A.M.A.* **81**:353.

BORMANN, R. VON. 1940. Hepatitis epidemica. *Ergeb. Inn. Med. Kinderheilk.* **58**:201.

CAPPS, R. B. and STOKES, J. 1952. Epidemiology of infectious hepatitis and problems of prevalence and control. *J.A.M.A.* **149**:557.

COCKAYNE, E. A. 1912. Catarrhal jaundice, sporadic and epidemic, and its relation to acute yellow atrophy of the liver. *Quart. J. Med.* **6**:1.

EICHENWALD, H. F. 1955. Viral hepatitis: Clinical, laboratory and public health aspects. Public Health Service Publication 435. Washington, D.C.: Department of Health, Education, and Welfare.

ELLIS, F. B. 1953. Infective hepatitis and arsenotherapy hepatitis as it occurred amongst naval personnel in Portsmouth during the 1939–45 war. *Am. J. Hyg.* **51**:145–56.

EPPINGER, H. 1922. Die pathogenese des Ikterus. *Verhandl. Deut. Ges. Inn. Med.* **34**:15.

EXPERT COMMITTEE ON HEPATITIS. 1953. Technical Report Ser. No. 62. Geneva: World Health Organization.

FINDLAY, G. M., MacCALLUM, F. O., and MURGATROYD, F. 1939. Observations bearing on the aetiology of infective hepatitis (so-called epidemic catarrhal jaundice). *Trans. Roy. Soc. Trop. Med. Hyg.* **32**:575.

FLAUM, A., MALMROS, H., and PERSSON, E. 1926. Eine nosocomiale Ikterus-Epidemie. *Acta Med. Scand.* Suppl. 16.

FOLLEY, F. E. and GUTHEIM, R. N. 1956. Serum hepatitis following dental procedures: A presentation of 15 cases including 3 fatalities. *Ann. Int. Med.* **45**:369.

FOX, J. P., MANSO, C., PENNA, H. A., and PARA, M. 1942. Observations on the occurrence of icterus in Brazil following vaccination against yellow fever. *Am. J. Hyg.* **36**:68.

GILES, J. P., LIEBHABER, H., KRUGMAN, S., and LATTIMER, C. 1964. Early viremia and viruria and infectious hepatitis. *J. Virol.* **24**:107.

HAVENS, W. P., JR. 1954. Review of attempts to test for immune bodies produced against the hepatitis agent. In *Symposium on the laboratory propagation and detection of the agent of hepatitis.* National Academy of Sciences, National Research Council, Publication 322, p. 93. Washington, D.C.

———. 1963. Viral hepatitis, *Ann. Rev. Med.* **14**:57.

HAVENS, W. P., JR. and PAUL, J. R. 1965. *Infectious and serum hepatitis.* In: *Viral and rickettsial infections in man,* eds. W. P. HORSFALL and I. TAMM, 4th ed. Philadelphia: J. B. Lippincott Co.

HAVENS, W. P., JR., WARD, R., DRILL, V. A., and PAUL, J. R. 1944. Experimental production of hepatitis by feeding icterogenic materials. *Proc. Soc. Exp. Biol. Med.* **57**:206.

Hepatitis Surveillance Reports. 1961–65. U.S. Public Health Service. Atlanta, Ga.: Communicable Disease Center.

HILLIS, W. D. 1961. An outbreak of infectious hepatitis among chimpanzee handlers at a United States Air Force Base. *Am. J. Hyg.* **73**:316.

HORSTMANN, D. M., HAVENS, W. P., and DEUTSCH, J. 1947. Infectious hepatitis in childhood, *J. Pediat.* **30**:381.

KRUGMAN, S., GILES, J. P., WARD, R., BODANSKY, O., and JACOBS, A. M. 1959. Infectious hepatitis. Detection of virus during the incubation period and in clinically inapparent infection. *New Engl. J. Med.* **261**:729.

KUH, C. and WARD, W. E. 1950. Occupational virus hepatitis. An apparent hazard for medical personnel. *J.A.M.A.* **143**:631.

LIAO, S., BERG, F. P., and BOUCHARD, R. J. 1954. Epidemiology of infectious hepatitis in an urban group. *Yale J. Biol. Med.* **26**:512.

LÜRMAN, A. 1885. Eine Icterusepidemie. *Berliner klin. Wochschr.* p. 24.

MELNICK, J. L. 1956. *Water-borne epidemic of infectious hepatitis in India. Proceedings International Conference on Hepatitis, Detroit.* Boston: Little, Brown & Co.

MIRICK, G. S., WARD, R., and McCOLLUM, R. W. 1962. Gamma globulin in the control of hepatitis following blood transfusion. *Vox Sanguinis* **7**:125.

MURRAY, R., DIEFENBACH, W. C. L., GELLER, H., LEONE, N. C., and RATNER, F. 1955. The problem of reducing the danger of serum hepatitis from blood and blood products. *New York J. Med.* **55**:1145.

NEEFE, J. R., *et al.* 1954. Carriers of hepatitis virus in the blood and viral hepatitis in whole blood recipients. 1. Studies in donors suspected as carriers of hepatitis virus and sources of post-transfusion viral hepatitis. *J.A.M.A.* **154**:1066.

NEEFE, J. R. and STOKES, J. 1945. An epidemic of infectious hepatitis apparently due to a water-borne agent. *J.A.M.A.* **128**:1063.

NEEFE, J. R., STOKES, J., JR., and REINHOLD, J. G. 1945. Oral administration to volunteers of feces from patients with homologous serum hepatitis and infectious (epidemic) hepatitis. *Am. J. Med. Sci.* **210**:29.

PARR, L. W. 1945. Host variation in the manifestation of disease, with particular reference to homologous serum jaundice in the Army of the United States. *Med. Ann. Dist. Columbia* **14**:443–49.

PAUL, J. R. and GARDNER, H. T. 1950. Endemiological aspects of hepatitis in U.S. troops in Germany, 1946–1950. *Am. J. Med.* **8**:565–80.

————. 1960. Viral Hepatitis. In *Medical Department, U.S. Army. Preventive medicine in World War II. Communicable diseases transmitted through contact or by unknown means.* Vol. V, pp. 411–62. Washington, D.C. U.S. Government Printing Office.

PAUL, J. R., HAVENS, W. P., JR., SABIN, A. B., and PHILIP, C. B. 1945. Transmission experiments in serum jaundice and infectious hepatitis, *J.A.M.A.* **128**:911.

QUINCKE, A. 1903. Icterus epidemicus in diseases of the liver, pancreas, and suprarenal capsules. In *Nothnagel's encyclopedia of practical medicine,* translated by ALFRED STENGEL. Vol. 8, p. 500. Philadelphia: W. B. Saunders.

RICH, A. R. 1930. The pathogenesis of the forms of jaundice. *Bull. Johns Hopkins Hosp.* **47**:338.

SAWYER, W. A., MEYER, K. F., EATON, M. D., BAUER, J. R., PUTNAM, P., and SCHWENTKER, F. F. 1944. Jaundice in army personnel in the western region of the United States and its relation to vaccination against yellow fever. *Am. J. Hyg.* **39**:337–430; **40**:35–107.

SHERMAN, I. L. and EICHENWALD, H. F. 1956. Viral hepatitis: Descriptive epidemiology based on morbidity and mortality statistics. *Ann. Int. Med.* **44**:1049.

SMITH, B. F. 1950. Occurrence of hepatitis in recently tattooed service personnel. *J.A.M.A.* **144**:1074.

STOKES, J., JR. 1962. The control of viral hepatitis. *Am. J. Med.* **32**:729.

STOKES, J., JR., BERK, J. E., MALAMUT, L. L., DRAKE, M. E., BARONDESS, J. A., BASHE, W. J., WOLMAN, I. J., FARQUHAR, J. D., BEVAN, B., DRUMMOND, R. J., MAYCOCK, W. D'A., CAPPS, R. B., and BENNETT, A. M. 1954. The carrier state in viral hepatitis. *J.A.M.A.* **154**:1059.

TRUMBULL, M. L. and GREINER, D. J. 1951. Homologous serum jaundice: An occupational hazard to medical personnel. *J.A.M.A.* **145**:965.

TUCKER, C. B. and FARREL, R. P. 1954. An outbreak of infectious hepatitis apparently transmitted through water. *Southern Med. J.* **47**:732.

VOEGT, H. 1942. Zur Aetiologie der Hepatitis epidemica. *München. Med. Wochschr.* **89**:76.

WARD, R. and KRUGMAN, S. 1958. *Endemic hepatitis in an institution. Proceedings International Conference on Hepatitis, Detroit.* Boston: Little, Brown & Co.

WARD, R. and KRUGMAN, S. 1961. Viral hepatitis. *DM* June.

WARD, R., KRUGMAN, S., and GILES, J. P. 1960. Etiology and prevention of infectious hepatitis. *Postgrad. Med.* **28**:12.

WARD, R., KRUGMAN, S., GILES, J. P., JACOBS, A. M., and BODANSKY, O. 1958. Infectious hepatitis. Studies of its natural history and prevention. *New Engl. J. Med.* **258**:207.

WEWALKA, F. 1953. Zur Epidemiologie des Ikterus bei der antisyphilitischen Behandlung. *Schweiz. Z. Allgem. Path. Bakteriol.* **16**:307–12.

CHAPTER XVIII

Arthropod-borne Virus Infections

Applied to virus infections, the term arthropod-borne [1] might be defined merely as the mechanical transfer of virus from one host to another by an insect, but the term implies more than that; namely, that the virus survives for long periods within the arthropod-host, during which time it may increase in amount. Besides insects, these viruses infect a number of hosts, such as birds, even reptiles, and various mammals including man. The infection may depend upon a cycle in which viruses travel from insect to vertebrate and back to insect. The maintenance of such an ecologic pattern depends upon balanced interrelationships, involving the environmental setting, climate, the viruses, and appropriate hosts—arthropod and otherwise—one or more of which may act as an interepidemic reservoir of the virus.

Many viral agents that cause human and animal diseases attack the central nervous system. In some diseases, this occurs very rarely in the course of an infection; in others, it happens frequently, and the viral agent has been termed neurotropic. From the large family of virus infections, we have singled out a group of viruses that are arthropod-borne, largely neurotropic and that have received considerable attention from students of epidemiology.

Some of the members of this huge family of viruses are more closely related antigenically than others. This has allowed a provisional classification into 20 groups or more (A, B, C, and so forth). I have arbitrarily chosen some of the better-known

---

[1] The term arthropod-borne viruses has been conveniently shortened to arboviruses.

members of group A and B, to be listed below, together with the major geographical sites where they are located. These are:

Group A:

    Eastern equine encephalomyelitis (EEE).........United States
    Western equine encephalomyelitis (WEE)........North America
    Venezuelan encephalomyelitis (VEE).............North coast of
                   South America

Group B:

    St. Louis encephalitis (STL)....................United States
    Japanese encephalitis (JE) [2]....................Japan, Korea
    West Nile fever (WN).........................Africa and Middle
                   East
    Murray Valley encephalitis (MVE)..............Australia
    Russian spring-summer (tick-borne) encephalitis
      (RSSE).................................Russia, Siberia

Other arboviruses which are regarded as less neurotropic for man than those mentioned above will not be considered at this time. They include yellow fever, dengue, and a long list of agents most of which have been isolated during the past two decades in Africa, India, and South America.

Historical Note

This story began, perhaps, in Japan, where periodic epidemics of encephalitis have been recorded since the late nineteenth century. These epidemics were extensive and more or less unique for that time, often causing thousands of deaths. In all probability they represented examples of what was later to be identified as the mosquito-borne viral infection of Japanese encephalitis.

Another form of encephalomyelitis, similar to that in Japan, appeared in Australia for a brief span from 1917 to 1919. Designated as the Australian X disease, it apparently disappeared as suddenly and mysteriously as it had first appeared. A generation later, however, it cropped up again in southeastern

[2] Originally designated as Japanese B encephalitis to distinguish it from what the Japanese chose to call the A type of encephalitis (Von Economo's disease). The letter *B* has been dropped from the name recently by some authors.

Australia and this time was classified and enrolled as another member of the B group of arthropod-borne virus infections and given a new name—Murray Valley encephalitis. It was another example of the peculiar epidemiologic features of this family of diseases; one member may appear in epidemic form and then disappear for twenty years or more.

In the United States the first great outbreak of summer encephalitis occurred in St. Louis, Missouri, in 1933, and there has seldom been an urban epidemic of this size in North America since. From the cases in this St. Louis epidemic a virus was isolated, designated later as St. Louis encephalitis virus, (STL) which, together with the previously isolated Japanese encephalitis virus, indicated that there might be a new family of viruses causing somewhat similar diseases (Webster and Fite 1933). Shortly thereafter, about 1937, in Russia and Siberia, a very widespread and serious form of tick-borne viral encephalitis was recognized and given a name reflecting its seasonal occurrence—Russian spring-summer encephalitis; western and eastern varieties are now recognized (Smorodintsev 1954).

But at this point we must retrace our steps and explain that some viral encephalitides had been recognized in animals before they were recognized in man (Casals 1957). In 1930, a disease known to be present in Scotland for more than a century, that attacked the nervous system of sheep, and called louping ill, was shown to be due to a virus. In the United States two of the varieties, western and eastern equine encephalomyelitis, were first identified as viral diseases of horses, the former in 1931 (Meyer, Haring, and Howitt 1931). It was thought at this time that they belonged wholly in the field of veterinary medicine. But a most revealing discovery came in the summer of 1938, when it was found in New England that the host range of eastern equine encephalomyelitis (EEE) virus was not limited to horses, but could also include man. In fact, EEE virus gives rise to a serious form of human encephalitis. Shortly thereafter, the same was demonstrated for western equine encephalomyelitis (WEE), which in 1941 and subsequently, was recognized in the western United States and Canada in epidemic and sporadic form. In the

U.S. the disease has been constantly recognized in horses (Communicable Disease Reports 1955–64). Epidemics and sporadic cases of WEE have been fairly prevalent in man in the entire western half of the country; the same is true for STL in almost the entire United States, and human epidemics of EEE have occurred in Massachusetts and New Jersey.

ECOLOGY

Outstanding features of these illnesses are that many cases of infection escape clinical recognition, and that so many involve extrahuman hosts. It now seems clear that both groups A and B of the viruses listed on page 222 (except RSSE, which is tickborne) are transmitted largely by mosquitoes and that the primary cycle in nature is one of mosquito to bird to mosquito, or mosquito to small mammal to mosquito. When domestic and large mammals and man occasionally fall into this arthropod cycle, it seems to be accidental since the suspected vectors seem to prefer feeding on favorite species. Nevertheless, infection of a wide variety of mammalian species occurs. In the case of Japanese encephalitis this includes—besides man and horses—dogs, swine, sheep, and goats, in which the disease may be mild, although evidence of infection can be demonstrated by serologic means.

For these infections to maintain themselves within a given geographical area, certain conditions must be present. (1) There must be a susceptible arthropod vector in which the virus can multiply sufficiently to be transmitted in infectious dosage during the feeding procedure. (2) Susceptible mammals or birds must always have a relatively rapid population turnover, so that enough susceptibles are present each year in which the virus can multiply to produce a viremia of sufficient titer to infect a feeding arthropod vector. (3) There must be a means of carryover of the virus through nonepidemic seasons of the year.

Over and above the arthropod means of transmission, there may be other subsidiary and special mechanisms, such as milkborne cases, in which man drinks milk from goats bitten by ticks and thus infected with RSSE virus. Such milk-borne RSSE infections have occurred on a fairly large scale in Russia and Siberia. Another example of extra-arthropod spread is the direct transmission of eastern equine encephalomyelitis from bird to bird, which has occurred in pheasants being reared artificially in pens. A third, and happily very rare, situation is that of accidental (laboratory) infection in man.

EPIDEMIC ASPECTS IN MAN

Three or four of the members of groups A and B will be chosen to illustrate the epidemiologic behavior of these viral infections in man, although it is obvious that each member may have certain features not characteristic of the group as a whole. Data will be used from a single early epidemic of western equine encephalomyelitis, which seemed to start in the province of Manitoba, Canada.

This outbreak began early in August, 1941, and lasted until mid-September. The epidemic eventually covered a very large area, of which the province of Manitoba was but a part, extending into two neighboring states in the United States and into the adjacent province of Saskatchewan in Canada. Within the whole area, about 2,300 human cases were recorded during the summer season, 509 of which occurred in Manitoba, with a case fatality rate of 15.3 per cent.

Attack rates were lower in the urban population of the principal city of Winnipeg than in other districts (see Table 6).

TABLE 6

DISTRIBUTION OF CASES OF WESTERN EQUINE ENCEPHALOMYELITIS (WEE) IN THE PROVINCE OF MANITOBA, CANADA IN 1941

District	Population (1941 Census)	Cases	Rate per 100,000
Urban: Winnipeg	217,994	108	49
Suburban: south of Winnipeg	73,374	58	79
Remainder of province	431,079	343	79

Data from Donovan and Bowman, 1942.

These data indicated either a higher exposure rate in rural or semirural areas or a more immune urban population. Serological surveys demonstrated that it was the former situation that was responsible for the rural prevalence of this insect-borne infection. In other words, the higher rural rates were in all probability associated with living or working conditions that caused the rural population to be more exposed to mosquitoes than urban residents.

AGE AND SEX DISTRIBUTION

Estimates of age-specific rates per 100,000 for males and females indicated that in this large epidemic approximately 81 per cent of the patients were twenty or over, with particularly high rates in the older age groups. At all ages the male cases outnumbered the female, except among infants. Actually, of the 509 cases in the Manitoba epidemic, 70 per cent were males.

Donovan and Bowman (1942) stated their belief that, in this previously nonimmune population, the high attack rates in male individuals over twenty, particularly those in rural areas, could be explained by the fact that these adults represented the most vulnerable segment of the population—laborers in an agricultural district where irrigation was practiced and therefore where mosquitoes were more numerous than in other areas. It might be mentioned, however, that as World War II was still in progress many more older men apparently were engaged in work connected with the harvest than usual.

The age distribution in this, an isolated epidemic of WEE, is given as a special example and is one that would not necessarily occur elsewhere. In Japan, for instance, where the clinical infection of Japanese encephalitis, both epidemic and endemic, has periodically been much more common and the exposure rate is high, the adult population has a higher degree of immunity. Thus Japanese encephalitis becomes automatically a children's disease because they are the only susceptibles. This tends to push the clinical disease into lower age brackets, with encephalitis rates as high as 117 per 100,000 in the ages between six and ten years, in contrast to lower rates in adults.

The actual ratios of clinically diagnosed cases to subclinical or inapparent infections by various members of this family of infections and in various epidemics varies greatly. If the disease behaves as does Japanese encephalitis, only a small fraction of the total infections are overt, recognized clinically, and labeled. Indeed the ratio of cases of overt encephalitis to inapparent infection may be 1:90 or 1:99.

The widespread distribution of the infection in Japan makes it easier to determine serologically the age prevalence of antibodies so that a successful mapping of the geographical and historical frequency can be made. In the region around Tokyo, for instance, and around the Inland Sea, almost 90–100 per cent of the natives over thirty years of age possess neutralizing antibodies.

TYPES OF INSECT VECTORS AND HOST RANGE

By and large, culex mosquitoes have proved to be important insect vectors known to harbor and transmit this group of viruses. *Culex tarsalis* and *C. pipiens* are the most prominent for St. Louis and western equine encephalomyelitis virus; *Culiseta melanura* for eastern equine encephalomyelitis; *C. tritaeniorhynchus* for Japanese encephalitis in Japan, and *C. univittatis* for West Nile virus infections in North Africa, to mention but a few.

The list of avian and mammalian hosts that may be infected differs from place to place and may depend upon the species preferences certain mosquitoes have in their individual feeding habits. Birds may be more important hosts than small mammals, and yet the latter have a suspected but not yet convincingly demonstrated importance in the maintenance of some endemic cycles. Usually the infection in the bird is not a serious illness, and the only way it can be demonstrated is by the detection of viremia and/or an appropriate rise of antibodies. Not infrequently such demonstrations can be made in the fledglings in the nest, which are both vulnerable, owing to lack of feathers, and susceptible. So it is during the nesting season that considerable activity in the mosquito-bird cycle is going on. For some species of birds, such as pheasants, an infection with one of these viruses, particularly eastern equine encephalomyelitis, may be very serious, especially when these birds are kept in pens and there is an opportunity for the sick pheasants to be attacked by their stronger pen mates. Mortality rates, ranging up to 75 per cent or higher, may result in individual pens. Under these circumstances, the virus is transmitted directly from bird to bird by means of pecking. This phenomenon may occur without any detectable evidence of the infection spreading to man (Liao 1955). In Connecticut, for instance, summer after summer EEE infections have been noted on several pheasant farms and occasionally in local mammalian (equine) hosts, but, although the virus is obviously present in the community, almost no human cases and no evidence of inapparent human infections have occurred over a period of many years (Jungherr and Wallis 1958).

In vertebrates, infection with most of these viruses is a brief event. Either the host succumbs or it survives through the marshaling of immunity mechanisms; in either event, the sojourn of the virus in the body and its accessibility to arthropods is short. In the arthropod vector the relationship is different. The viruses may produce no ill effect and remain in the arthropod throughout its natural life. Insects fit the role of permanent hosts and reservoirs more nearly than do vertebrates.

The mere recovery of a virus of this group from an arthropod, or the presence of specific antibodies against the virus in a vertebrate host does not necessarily imply that either the arthropod or the vertebrate is involved in the cycle of transmitting the virus or maintaining it in the community. For the arthropod to be involved, it must be able to acquire and transmit the infection by a bite. Similarly, the vertebrate must not only be susceptible to infection by the bite of the infected arthropod, but the animal must also circulate sufficient virus in the blood after infection to infect in turn, a second arthropod vector. In other words, if the cycle is to be maintained, the degree of viremia must reach a titer that represents a dose capable of infecting a biting arthropod. The hypothetical cycle proposed by Taylor *et al.* (1956), which may operate in the maintenance of West Nile infections, is reproduced in Fig. 35. With many other arboviruses ticks may take the place of mosquitoes; in those which are mosquito-borne, small mammals (and even some reptiles) may occupy a place in the picture.

Two methods or a combination thereof may be used in the recognition or diagnosis of these viral infections, recalling the techniques used with poliomyelitis: (*a*) isolating and identifying

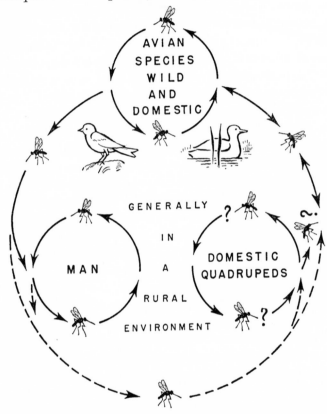

FIG. 35. Diagram illustrating hypothetical cycles of West Nile virus. Note that the complete cycle involving domestic quadrupeds is questioned. (Redrawn from Taylor et al., 1956. A study of the ecology of West Nile virus in Egypt. *Am. J. Trop. Med. Hyg.* **5:**579.)

the virus, and (*b*) testing for specific antibodies [3] to the virus in the blood of the suspected vertebrate host. The latter is useful for

[3] A variety of antibodies have been measured by different techniques: neutralizing, complement fixing, hemagglutination inhibiting and agar-gel methods are among those which have been used.

diagnosing an observed illness and for determining evidence of past infection. To diagnose an illness from antibody determinations, it is essential to have a blood specimen taken during the incipiency of the attack and a second specimen taken several weeks later. Generally an appropriate rise in antibodies with any of the approved tests, which occurs between these matched serum specimens is presumptive evidence that the virus antigen used in the test represents the agent responsible for the illness.

A word of caution should be expressed here regarding the specificity of the antibody reaction, for infection with one virus may stimulate antibodies to other antigenically related viruses. For example, Japanese encephalitis (JE), Murray Valley (MV), West Nile (WN), and Ntaya viruses, although sufficiently different to warrant individual names, may induce infection capable of stimulating heterologous antibodies common to the group. In certain areas of Egypt, for instance, it was found by Taylor *et al.* (1956) that about 8 per cent of the local human bloods would neutralize JE virus and about 34 per cent would neutralize Ntaya virus, but it was also found that all of the bloods that neutralized JE and nearly all that neutralized Ntaya also neutralized WN virus, which was the only virus that had been isolated locally from man, from birds, and from mosquitoes. Probably the JE and Ntaya viruses were not the local cause of these antibodies, and the response to JE and Ntaya has merely a broad or group antibody response. This observation has considerable bearing on interpretations of serological surveys from the standpoint of the specific arboviral infection involved.

THE SEROLOGIC APPROACH

For reasons just mentioned the optimal choice of an area for serologic survey of arboviral antibodies would be an area in which only one member of a given antigenic group was present. An example of this is in the northeastern corner of Africa, notably in Egypt and the Sudan, where West Nile virus infections are common and where other members of the Group B arboviruses are much less common. Taking advantage of this fact, Taylor and his colleagues mapped out the prevalence of various antibodies to WN virus. The resulting pattern was an index of infection that showed varying incidences with low, medium, and high rates in the Nile Delta, high rates in Cairo and Upper Egypt, and medium rates in the Sudan (Table 7). Measured by the neutralization test these data also indicated roughly the ages when people acquired this infection in this particular area, in the early 1950's.

TABLE 7

WEST NILE VIRUS-NEUTRALIZING ANTIBODIES IN THE INDIGENOUS HUMAN POPULATIONS OF EGYPT AND THE SUDAN, SUMMARIZED ACCORDING TO REGION [a]

REGION	NEUTRALIZATION								
	0+14 YEARS			15+ YEARS			ALL AGES		
	Number [b]	+	Percentage	Number [b]	+	Percentage	Number [b]	+	Percentage
Delta (Lower Egypt):									
Nonendemic area.	134	3	2	206	80	39	340	83	24
Transitional area.	49	8	16	56	41	73	105	49	47
Endemic area....	171	120	70	220	208	95	391	328	84
Cairo..........	15	4	27	92	60	65	107	64	60
Upper Egypt.......	103	65	63	121	107	88	224	172	77
Egypt, total.....	472	200	42	695	496	71	1167	696	60
Sudan............	146	41	28	204	98	48	350	139	40
Grand total....	618	241	39	899	594	66	1517	835	55

[a] Data, slightly modified, from Taylor *et al.*, 1956.
[b] Number of bloods tested.

Other important uses of the neutralization test have been the detection of antibodies and measurement of their various patterns in certain local vertebrate hosts such as mammals and birds in the endemic area. Table 8 shows the percentages at which neutralizing antibodies were demonstrated in these species, ranging from zero in the rat to 86 per cent in the horse. As a control for these studies, the sera from fifteen horses and sheep from England were examined. None of these sera neutralized WN virus. The sera from fourteen horses were also obtained from Brazil, and of these, two neutralized the virus. Other viruses antigenically related to WN are known to exist in Brazil, however, and may have accounted for the positive reactions. Positive tests were found in avian sera collected in the endemic area from almost all the local species of birds, both domesticated and wild. Percentages ranged from 14 per cent in domestic ducks to 65 per cent in the crow. Twenty-four chickens were imported from the United States as controls; none of their sera neutralized WN virus.

TABLE 8

WEST NILE VIRUS-NEUTRALIZATION TESTS ON SERA FROM MAMMALS AND AVIAN SPECIES FROM AN ENDEMIC AREA IN LOWER EGYPT

SPECIES	NUMBER TESTED	POSITIVE Number	POSITIVE Per-centage
Mammals:			
Camel...............................	9	7	78
Cow..................................	36	6	17
Donkey..............................	15	7	47
Gamoose (water buffalo).................	188	135	72
Goat.................................	49	1	2
Horse................................	14	12	86
Sheep................................	64	15	23
Rat..................................	43	0	..
Bat..................................	48	4	8
Total mammals.....................	466	187	40
Avian species:			
Chicken (domestic).....................	24	4	16
Rebleedings on previous negatives.......	15	2	13
Crow (*Corvus corone sardonius*)............	163	102	65
Duck (domestic).......................	14	2	14
Dove (*Streptopelia senegalensis senegalensis*) .	8	2	25
Goose (domestic).......................	29	6	27
Heron (*Bubulcus ibis ibis*)...............	65	18	28
Hoopoe (*Upupa epops major*).............	5	0	..
Kestrel (*Falco tinnunculus*)..............	3	3	..
Kite (*Milvus migrans aegyptius*)..........	1	1	..
Pigeon (domestic)......................	59	15	25
Sparrow (*Passer domesticus*).............	26	11	42
Quail (*Coturnix c. coturnix*)..............	8	0	..
Total avian species..................	420	170	40
Grand total........................	886	357	40

Data from Taylor *et al.*, 1956.

VIRUS ISOLATIONS FROM MOSQUITOES

Added to the evidence of past infection, the isolation of virus from locally caught mosquitoes is a most important aspect of this type of ecologic study. Details of this will not be reviewed here, for it is a special field of its own. In the Egyptian study, WN virus was recovered during the summer months for three successive years—1952, 1953, and 1954—in which mosquito collections were made. Each isolation represented many mosquitoes, and the rate of specimens that were positive was about 0.015 per cent.

This group of diseases falls into the pattern of infections that have a complex ecologic cycle, with the assumed purpose of the survival of the parasite. The situation reminds us of other, perhaps better-known, parasites that pass through several species of hosts such as the trichina worm or the fish or dog tapeworms. These cycles, besides being complex, do not always follow a fixed epidemiologic pattern. Man often seems to be an outsider as far as the main cycle is concerned, but for an understanding of the situation, the whole complex pattern should be known.

In the past six or eight years the number of arboviruses has enormously increased so that literally scores have been recently identified. Some are the causes of serious disease such as the hemorrhagic fevers, which have cropped up in the Asian continent and South America, and many have practically no significance for man. The story is far from completion.

BIBLIOGRAPHY

BAWEL, M. B., DEUEL, R. E., MATUMOTO, M., and SABIN, A. B. 1950. Status and significance of inapparent infection with the virus of Japanese B encephalitis in Japan in 1946. *Am. J. Hyg.* **51**:1.

CARTER, H. R. 1931. Yellow fever: *An epidemiological and historical study of its place of origin.* Baltimore: Williams & Wilkins Co.

CASALS, J. 1957. The arthropod-borne group of animal viruses. *Trans. N.Y. Acad. Sci., Ser. II* **19**:219.

COMMUNICABLE DISEASE REPORTS. Surveillance of arthropod-borne encephalitis in the United States (1955–1959). U.S. Department of Health, Education, and Welfare. Atlanta, Ga.: Public Health Service.

DONOVAN, C. R. and BOWMAN, M. 1942. Some epidemiological features of poliomyelitis and encephalitis, Manitoba, 1941. *Can. Public Health J.* **33**:246.

GAJDUSEK, D. C. and ROGERS, N. G. 1955. Specific serum antibodies to infectious disease agents in Tarahumara Indian adolescents of Northwestern Mexico. *Pediatrics* **16**:819.

JUNGHERR, E. L. and WALLIS, R. C. 1958. Investigation of eastern equine encephalomyelitis. I. General aspects. *Am. J. Hyg.* **67**:1.

LIAO, S. J. 1955. Eastern equine encephalitis in Connecticut: A serological survey of pheasant farmers. *Yale J. Biol. Med.* **27**:287.

MEYER, K. F., HARING, C. M., and HOWITT, B. 1931. The etiology of epizootic encephalomyelitis of horses in the San Joaquin Valley, 1930. *Science* **74**:227–28.

SCHLESINGER, R. W. 1952. The seasonal arthropod-borne virus encephalitis. In *Medical monographs,* ed. W. W. BEAN. Baltimore: Williams & Wilkins Co.

SMORODINSEV, A. A. (ed.). 1954. *Neurotropic virus infections.* Leningrad: Medgiz.

STRODE, G. K. (ed.). 1951. *Yellow fever.* New York: McGraw-Hill Book Co.

TAYLOR, R. M., WORK, T. H., HURLBURT, H. S., and RIZK, F. 1956. A study of the ecology of West Nile virus in Egypt. *Am. J. Trop. Med. Hyg.* **5**:579.

WEBSTER, L. T. and FITE, G. L. 1933. A virus encountered in the study of material from cases of encephalitis in the St. Louis and Kansas City epidemics of 1933. *Science* **78**:463.

WORK, T. H. and SHAH, K. V. 1956. Serological diagnosis of Japanese B type of encephalitis in North Arcot district of Madras State, India, with epidemiological notes. *Indian J. Med. Sci.* **10**:582.

CHAPTER XIX

Ischemic Heart Disease

Ischemic heart disease (IHD), which gives rise to the more commonly known manifestations of angina pectoris and coronary occlusion, has been chosen for review not only because it is an important twentieth century disease, but because the chances are that at least some of the puzzles that obscure its pathogenesis may eventually be explained by the study of its epidemiology (White 1957). Indeed, in the past fifteen years epidemiological studies in ischemic heart disease have been applied effectively with increasing frequency, and literature in this field has grown to such proportions that it will be impossible in this brief chapter to be comprehensive or even adequate. One feature deserving mention is that field studies seem to have gained ascendancy recently over those formerly derived from biostatistical analyses of mortality statistics.

It is fair to speak of IHD or coronary occlusion as a relatively "new" disease. Only since the 1920's has it become widely recognized as a common cardiac disease liable to kill important indviduals at the height of their business careers or wage-earning capacity. This has placed special, perhaps artificial, emphasis upon it, but at the same time it has vastly stimulated the interest of clinicians and health officials. Life insurance companies have long had a special interest in it. Such interest began when the diagnosis of coronary occlusion became generally acceptable in the early 1930's. Since then cases have been recognized with increasing frequency in the United States, and this is probably true of certain other countries. This recognition, in turn, has had a profound influence upon its recorded incidence.

Ischemic Heart Disease

In this country, ischemic heart disease is often referred to as public health problem No. 1. To appreciate its magnitude, for instance, its incidence, according to the survey made in middle aged men in Framingham, Massachusetts was a little more than one per cent per year (Dawber and Kannel 1961).

Diagnosis and Terminology

As with other cardiac diseases, the diagnosis of coronary occlusion may be lost in a morass of terms, of which arteriosclerotic heart disease, chronic myocardial disease, and coronary thrombosis are examples. Such loose terms may or may not include IHD or coronary occlusion. Another that nearly always implies coronary occlusion is myocardial infarction. A much more venerable term is angina pectoris. Angina pectoris, however, is actually a symptomatic diagnosis, used in those cases in which the patient often, but not always, suffers from characteristic pain and discomfort in the chest. It is characteristic of disease of the coronary arteries and should not be used as an equivalent of the term coronary occlusion, for the circumstances under which the two conditions arise are not always the same. Figure 36 shows four common diagnostic terms, some of which might imply the presence of fatal coronary artery disease that were employed over a twenty-five-year period in the second quarter of the twentieth century.

It is important to indicate that the pathogenesis of coronary occlusion may stem from at least two different sources. Thus closure of the coronary arteries, atherosclerosis and acute thrombosis, may participate as separate factors. Atherosclerosis, or atheroma, is a different entity from arteriosclerosis, and the two terms should be defined. Arteriosclerosis has been ascribed to vascular aging. The arterial changes associated with the involutional processes of aging do not often occlude the lumen of vessels. The changes due to arteriosclerosis occur within the muscular and elastic elements of the vessel wall, which are replaced in the median layer by collagen and, to a lesser extent, calcium is deposited there. Atherosclerosis, on the other hand, appears to be a metabolic disease, the lesions consisting of

236

patchy cholesterolosis and scarring of the intimal or inner layer of the vessel wall that have a tendency to extend into the median or muscular wall. The other factor, the acute thrombosis that actually occludes the lumen, may well develop on mural atheroma, but the two processes are not the same. Unfortunately little is known about the nature of intravascular thrombosis, and this

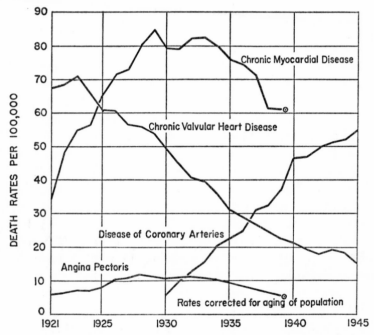

Fɪɢ. 36. Trends in diagnostic terminology in recording heart disease, 1920–45, in the United States. The chart depicts standardized death rates per 100,000 industrial policy holders of the Metropolitan Life Insurance Company. Graphs indicate how changing nomenclature has, in part at least, affected these rates. (From *Studies in heart disease*. 1946. New York: Metropolitan Life Insurance Co.)

might also be said about the true nature of atheroma formation. The latter often does narrow the lumen. It is far more common in the population than occlusive disease and was found to be extraordinarily prevalent in United States soldiers, mostly in their twenties, who were fatal battle casualties in the Korean War (Enos *et al.* 1953).

Historically, although angina pectoris was recognized as a clinical entity and given that name by Heberden in 1768, one of the first to recognize coronary artery disease as the cause of the lesions that give rise to the symptoms of angina pectoris was Edward Jenner, of smallpox vaccination fame. Among early cases was that of John Hunter in 1773, who had an attack at the age of 45,—and described the symptoms himself. He was to suffer subsequent anginal attacks but lived 20 years more. At his autopsy, the coronary arteries had the appearance of "bony tubes" (Ryle 1928).

For many years, however, the correct view of the cause of anginal attacks or of sudden cardiac deaths remained a mystery. Often they were ascribed to "acute indigestion" and this concept lasted for more than a century. That coronary occlusion may be a cause of sudden death came largely from the observations of James B. Herrick, an American physician. He first reported this finding in 1912 and again in a second communication seven years later. By 1920 practitioners and internists were apparently ready to consider the new idea. In any event the diagnosis of coronary occlusion became generally acceptable in the 1930's, and subsequently cases have been recognized with increasing frequency. The idea that diet might have something to do with atherosclerosis seems to have developed slowly, although it had been raised by Anitschow's early experimental work, which dates back to 1914.

Methods of Estimating the Prevalence of Coronary Artery Disease

Most of the early information about the over-all frequency of fatal coronary artery disease has been obtained from large-scale mortality statistics assembled by life insurance companies, health departments, or special surveys. These statistics suffer from the fact that among recorded diagnoses *arteriosclerotic heart disease* has been and still is a popular one; it may or may not include coronary artery disease.[1] The crude mortality rates for this catch-

---

[1] Coronary artery disease may be a localized manifestation of generalized atherosclerosis, and as such the extracardiac manifestations may overshadow the clinical picture when it comes to the terminal diagnosis.

all are not particularly meaningful, and, besides being judged in the light of the looseness of the diagnostic terms, they should be weighed with other variables.

Since the reporting of ischemic heart disease as a distinct clinical entity has not yet become universal in the United States, facts about its prevalence in this country usually have to be gathered from special surveys conducted by the U.S. Public Health Service, or from sickness surveys conducted by special teams of investigators. In the most recent National Health Survey covering the years 1960 to 1962, the prevalence of coronary heart disease among males and females, aged 18–79 was recorded as 2.8 per cent. If suspect cases were included, this figure would be much higher.

Some of these smaller morbidity surveys have proved to be of value in far more ways than the mere estimation of age-specific incidence rates. As an example one can cite the well-known survey carried out by Morris and his co-workers in an industrial population in England. This group determined rates of angina pectoris to be from less than 1 to about 7 per 1,000 in their population of 40–64-year-old employees of the London Transport Board. Among other important observations they made the point that the bus drivers in that population had an excess incidence of ischemic heart disease, age for age, in comparison to the bus conductors. The latter walk along the decks and climb and descend the stairs in contrast to the drivers who sit while at work. In other words, this survey yielded information that probably has bearing on pathogenesis. It led Morris (1964) to formulate his hypothesis to guide further investigations, indicating that: "Physical activity of work is a protection against coronary (ischaemic) heart disease. Men in physically active jobs have less ischaemic heart disease during middle age, what disease they have is less severe, and they develop it later than men in physically inactive jobs." This hypothesis has been challenged by some, supported by many others. Much more investigative work remains to be done in testing various aspects of the problem, but by and large, supporters of Morris' hypothesis outnumber its opponents.

In another more recent study by Kahn (1963), which was

made in an industrial population in the United States, this question of physical activity at work was pursued further. Kahn's survey was made under the auspices of the National Heart Institute at Bethesda, Maryland, and included two groups of middle-aged male employees of the Post Office in Washington, D.C., covering a total of 2,240 individuals. The physical activity involved in the work of these two groups differed, although they were of similar socioeconomic status. The basis of selection of

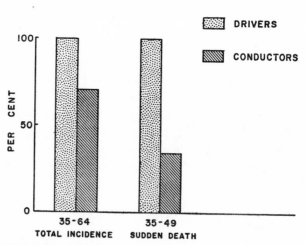

FIG. 37. Incidence of ischemic heart disease in London busmen, 1949–58. (Data from Morris, J. N., 1961, *Yale J. Biol. Med.* 34:359–69.)

these men was that they had been recruited between 1906 and 1940 and had remained in the Post Office for five years or more. The two groups consisted of letter carriers (postmen) required to do a considerable amount of walking, and postal clerks engaged in the more sedentary activity of sitting at a desk sorting letters. An analysis in terms of current service of the age-specific death rates for coronary heart disease in both groups indicated the clerk's rate to be 1.4 to 1.9 times as high as those of the letter carriers. Kahn's finding agrees with Morris' hypothesis that physical activity in middle-aged men is a prophylactic agent against early death from coronary heart disease.

In another survey in an industrial population in which it was more difficult to define jobs according to physical activity, Pell and D'Alonzo (1963) reviewed 1,356 cases of acute myocardial infarction that had occurred at the E. I. du Pont de Nemours and Company over a six year period ending in December, 1961. The employee population averaged 86,570; 75,573 were males, and the age range was from 25 to 64. The age-specific myocardial infarction rates are given in Table 9.

TABLE 9

Average Annual Age-specific Rates of Myocardial Infarction by Sex in the du Pont Company, 1956–61

AGE	No. of Cases		Rates per 1,000	
	Males	Females	Males	Females
25–29	1	0	0.02	0
30–34	14	1	0.19	0.09
35–39	71	2	0.96	0.18
40–44	166	0	2.45	0
45–49	276	3	4.78	0.38
50–54	340	5	7.93	0.87
55–59	280	6	10.36	1.74
60–64	183	8	10.86	4.14
All ages	1,331	25	3.02	0.32

Data from Pell and D'Alonzo, 1963. *J.A.M.A.* 185:831–38.

The rates listed in Table 9 again reflect the well-known higher risk with increasing age and the much higher risk in men than in women. These latter data are also consistent with the hypothesis that women lose their protection against coronary heart disease after the menopause.

It was also pointed out by these authors that in such a large company as du Pont there is a great diversity of occupations. Their efforts to classify these were resolved by dividing employees into five broad classifications based on salary levels and job responsibilities, level A being the highest and D the next to the lowest. The lowest was a large group of semi-skilled workers that they designated as "Wage roll." The descriptions of these categories are listed in Table 10.

241

Average, annual, age-specific incidence rates of myocardial infarction were computed for the various categories listed in Table 10. These rates appear in Fig. 38, which shows the highest to be among the foremen and clerical workers and the lowest, curiously enough, among the executives.

Pell and D'Alonzo also discuss certain risk factors estimated in their population that lead them to conclude that: hypertension increases the risk of myocardial infarction in all age groups included in their study but especially in men under 45 years of age; overweight was not associated with myocardial infarction

TABLE 10

JOB CLASSIFICATION BASED LARGELY ON SALARIES IN
THE DU PONT COMPANY

Category	No. of Employees	Description of Job
A	1,143	Executives, plant managers
B	10,241	Salesmen and research workers
C	10,631	Foremen, clerical supervisors, laboratory technicians
D	5,508	Clerical workers, some laborers and technicians
Wage roll	46,050	Semi-skilled workers and laborers

For age-specific incidence rates in categories see Fig. 38 (Data from Pell and D'Alonzo. 1963. *J.A.M.A.* **185**:831–38.)

between the ages of 45 and 64, but under 45 years of age the risk was increased when these conditions occurred jointly. Among men in the 45–64 age group who were both hypertensive and overweight, the estimated incidence rate was 5.6 times that of men with neither of these conditions. They further estimated the risk of myocardial infarction to be about two and one-half times as great among diabetics in this population than among non-diabetics.

On the other hand, it hardly can be said that this kind of study has led to universal agreement about the identification of factors contributing to the development of coronary heart disease. For instance, studies in California are not in particular agreement (Chapman *et al.* 1957). Furthermore, in a 5-year survey carried out from 1957 to 1963 in an industrial population in Chicago, on

242

about 2,000 male employees (aged 40–55) of the Western Electric Company, Paul *et al.* (1963) concluded that in this population, which in the years of observation had yielded an annual rate of coronary cases of about 0.9 per 1,000, there was "no relationship between body weight, blood sugar levels, lipoprotein lipase levels, or diet (other than coffee) and the development of coronary heart disease. Similarly there was no

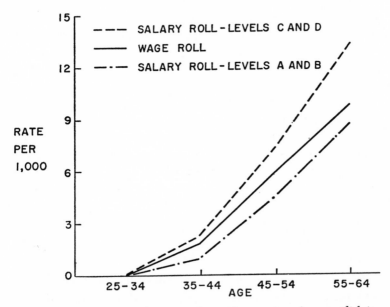

Fig. 38. Average annual age-specific incidence rates of myocardial infarction among employees of different wage or salary categories in the DuPont Company, to be compared with Table 10. (Data from Pell and D'Alonzo, 1963, *J. A. M. A.* 185:831.)

association with job type and no certain relation to physical activity off the job." It might be pointed out, however, that the age of the Chicago population (40–55) was younger than the du Pont population, if a comparison is to be drawn between these two studies.

Of the large number of other surveys, which have not been confined to industrial populations but have covered general populations, perhaps the best known is the Framingham survey, a field study made in Framingham, Massachusetts. This was instituted in 1950 under the direction of the National Heart Institute of the U.S. Public Health Service (Dawber and Kannel 1961, Dawber *et al.* 1962). In the intervening years it has produced a wealth of data, from which we will mention certain factors that the authors believe increase the risk of coronary heart disease in a general population. One factor involved the demonstration of high blood fats (lipemia) including high levels of serum cholesterol. This led the authors to conclude, as it has to many others before and since, that high levels of lipemia, in part perhaps the result of the ingestion of saturated fats, increase the risk of coronary heart disease. This risk, when measured in the male population, aged 30–49 at the time of entry, increased more than five fold from low to high levels of serum cholesterol. Another factor that applied to both males and females was an increase of blood pressure; another was overweight, but the authors felt that only those at the upper end of the relative weight scale have an added risk. When a combination of risk factors was present the chances of acquiring coronary heart disease were increased greatly.

As already mentioned, many such surveys could be quoted, and indeed the reason for describing so many already is that they illustrate the extensive use of epidemiological survey methods by clinicians and statisticians to solve some of the questions that still obscure the pathogenesis of IHD, a use that has proved to be singularly effective in the past decade. It will probably be more so in the future.

PATHOGENESIS

As has been obvious from opinions derived from the preceding discussions, a variety of factors seem to be involved in the pathogenesis of IHD. Hardly any one of them can be singled out as one to which special weight can be ascribed. Indeed multiple factors—some genetic, some representing personal habits, and some apparently environmental—may be contributory. Prominent among those mentioned have been hypertension, diabetes, obesity, the hyperlipemic values of cholesterol and triglycerides, curtailed physical activity, and cigarette smoking. These have all come in for their share of incrimination. Some of these will be taken up individually later in this chapter.

GENETIC TRAITS

It has been difficult to demonstrate with any degree of consistency traits that are truly hereditary. There have been examples of course of multiple cases in one family such as that described by Herapath and Perry (1930), but these seldom occur. Pertinent surveys include the work of Thomas and Hirschhorn (1955), which is part of a long-term analysis that Thomas and her coworkers have carried out on relatives of medical students at the Johns Hopkins Medical School; and those reviewed at the Symposium on Genetics and Epidemiology (1964). Thomas and Hirschhorn were at least able to determine that coronary artery disease was nearly four times as prevalent among siblings of individuals with coronary artery disease than among siblings of those without it. Such a clustering of cases within a given family does not necessarily reflect a hereditary predisposition. It well may be the result of parental or intrafamilial influences that shape the personal habits of a given family, such as over-eating, smoking, avoidance of physical activity, and so on.

RACE

It has been noted in the United States that Jews have a high rate of coronary occlusion, the Italians, a lower rate, and previously, the Negroes, had the lowest. This last statement should be qualified, however, for the increase of incidence in coronary rates in Negroes in the United States is becoming greater than that of whites. Again it is difficult to separate an actual inherited constitutional tendency to acquire this disease from racial habits or from situations intrinsic in the racial environment that may predispose to the development of coronary disease. For instance, an observation about this has come out of Israel that indicates pastoral immigrants to that nation have an extremely low incidence of this disease; but once these immigrants settled in Israel, and had lost their pastoral way of life, and changed their diets, the incidence of this disease became similar to that of the other inhabitants.

AGE AND SEX

Traditionally, myocardial infarction is a disease of middle-aged males, or perhaps those who are just beyond middle age. The age-specific rates listed by Pell and D'Alonzo in Table 9 give a good estimate as to the influence of age in that particular industrial population. Usually the highest prevalence has been recorded in the decade between 50 and 60, but the adjacent decades of life furnish large percentages of patients. In the compilation of age-specific rates it is important to know whether cases of angina (those indicating symptomatic evidences only of coronary heart disease) are included, and whether the data have been strictly limited to the ages at which first attacks occurred.

The rates listed in Table 9 reflect the risks with age as well as the much higher risk in men than in women. In various series of clinical cases covering all ages, 84 per cent of the subjects were males. The ratio of males to females in autopsied cases has been found to be similar—4.2 to 1. In a series of clinical cases collected in the age groups below forty, more than 95 per cent of the cases occurred in males. The data in Table 9, which reflect a sex differential within a special population, are also consistent with the belief that women lose their protection against coronary heart disease after the menopause. In fact, it is fairly well established that women who have had an artificial menopause have the same liability to the disease as men of the same age.

OBESITY

The experience of life insurance companies has long indicated that excess weight is accompanied by an increased mortality from cardiovascular diseases. We have already mentioned the conclusions by Dawber *et al.* (1962) of the Framingham team. Their investigations have shown the apparent effect of an increase in relative weight on coronary heart disease, but only those at the upper end of the relative weight scale have an added risk.

246

Albrink *et al.* (1962) have pursued this subject of overweight further, particularly as it concerned the development of an increase in serum lipids in the subjects they investigated. They arrived at the conclusion that, if the elevation of serum triglycerides is prognostic of coronary disease, then the man who has experienced a weight gain after the age of 25 has a special risk. In other words, if a child or adolescent who has been obese for some years or practically all his young life continues to be overweight in early adulthood, this individual does not suffer the same risk as the individual, who, for various reasons, begins to put on weight soon after he has reached 25.

An important consideration, which should be kept in mind when dealing with this kind of analysis of possible factors contributing directly or indirectly to the acquisition of coronary heart disease is that obesity and certain other features are seen frequently in diabetes.

PHYSICAL ACTIVITY

The idea that men who maintain a physically active life have less severe IHD than do those with sedentary occupations has already been discussed at length (see Fig. 37). To quote from Morris (1961–62): "The correlation between sedentary occupation and high rates of IHD have now been made in several countries including the United Kingdom, United States, Israel, Poland, Finland, Russia." Although in the California studies and the Chicago studies (Paul *et al.* 1963), there appears to be no relation to occupational activity at all, perhaps it is overwhelmed by other factors. Yet physically active workers seem to be healthier in middle age. Reduction of physical activity is one of the characteristic social changes of the present century, which automation promises to increase. Not all are in agreement with the above premise, however, and much further work remains to be done (Longstreet *et al.* 1962, Fox and Skinner, 1964).

HUMAN PHYSIQUE AND BODY TYPE

There have been repeated attempts to correlate coronary artery disease with body build, which in turn may be indirectly related to type of occupation, participation in athletic sports, aggressiveness in occupation, and so forth. By dividing male patients into three categories—endomorph, mesomorph, and ectomorph somatotypes (for a definition, see page 117)—Gertler and others (1954) have tried to determine whether men endowed with a particular kind of physique tend to acquire coronary disease more often than others. The method consisted of giving each individual a rating according to his degree of resemblance to one of the classical (Sheldon 1940) somatotypes. They found that among the coronary patients there was probably a predominance of the more massive and muscular forms of physique, in contrast to those of the control group that showed a wider distribution of body builds on the diagram.

HABITS, DIETS, AND WAYS OF LIFE

Individuals who find themselves in certain environments, whether they be occupational, social, or otherwise, often adopt the smoking, eating, and exercise habits of their friends and colleagues. This in turn may start special habits, which can soon become deeply rooted.

A relationship between cigarette smoking and coronary heart disease has long been suspected and yet often vehemently denied by some cardiologists. Only recently, however, has evidence accumulated, largely from epidemiological sources, that leaves little doubt that the excessive use of cigarettes and coronary heart disease are associated. This has been found in mortality data (Dorn 1959), and in many field surveys (Doyle *et al.* 1962, Smoking and Health 1964). The risk factor is not so pronounced as in cancer of the lung, but it is appreciable, especially in the mortality data.

It has been known for some time that the level of blood lipids can be lowered by reducing the amount of saturated fat in the diet. Thus blood cholesterol levels have long been singled out for study in this connection and considerable importance has been attached to them by some. Supplementing such views are many surveys that seem to illustrate in some populations, a correlation between a diet low in fats (with accompanying low blood cholesterol values) and a low mortality rate from coronary artery disease. For a geographic illustration of the influence of dietary habits on plasma lipid patterns and the incidence of atherosclerotic disease, one can examine and compare the data from different populations, as Malmros (1950) has done in Scandinavia. Italians, Spanish, Chinese, and Bantus from South Africa, who subsist on diets low in cholesterol and lipid, are said to be remarkably free of atherosclerotic disease. Perhaps a better type of epidemiological comparison would be the incidence of heart disease and the amount and kinds of fat consumed in Naples, Italy or in Ireland compared with Italian or Irish populations living in cities in the United States. Such comparisons are becoming available. In Norway, where fat consumption declined during the occupation of that country by the Germans in World War II, the incidence and mortality of IHD fell. After the war the normal Scandinavian diet was resumed and IHD rates soon increased. But Morris has pointed out that other influences came into the picture such as a reduction in total calories in the war diets with a corresponding fall in weight, more physical activity, and less cigarette smoking.

Current information derived from studies in patients and controls now reveals that the measure of blood lipids can keep track of fat consumption. Levels of triglycerides are a more sensitive measure than those of cholesterol. Data from Albrink's group indicate that although 46 per cent of men with coronary disease had elevated blood cholesterol levels as compared with 26 per cent in the control group, 82 per cent of the patients and 36 per cent of the controls had elevated triglyceride levels. These observations, and theories drawn from them, do not, however, justify the idea that the problem of fat consumption and the level of blood lipids is as simple as it may sound.

OCCUPATION

For more than a score of years it has been pointed out that farmers and laborers seem to be less prone to coronary atherosclerosis than foremen of work gangs or professional men such as physicians and lawyers. This is a lead that needs more research. It may well be that a number of factors are operative and that the demands of certain occupations, resulting in a sedentary life, are at the same time responsible for an excessive nervous strain. The hypothetical protection against coronary artery disease provided by work with physical activity must be clearly differentiated from brief periods of exercise—a game of golf or tennis once a month—and that experienced in shoveling snow or running for a train by a man not used to it.

HYPERTENSION

The presence of hypertension by itself or in combination with one or more of the risk factors considered in this chapter deserves mention. Nearly all those who have studied it in connection with the prevalence and/or the incidence of coronary artery disease have come to the conclusion that it does represent an appreciable risk factor, and when it occurs in combination with obesity the risk is greatly increased.

Conclusion

In summary, therefore, current theories of IHD etiology indicate that it is not concerned with aging alone but with certain incapacities on the part of some people to handle what they may have heretofore considered normal ways of life. I believe that the pathogenesis of IHD remains complex, since coronary occlusion and coronary atheroma have different causes, and both may be required for IHD to develop. These cannot be disposed of glibly in terms of consumption of saturated fat, lack of physical activity, or nervous strain.

Furthermore, it would appear that the epidemiologic approach may be peculiarly valuable in the study of coronary artery disease, which, although still in its infancy, holds promise for determining the frequency of this condition in certain populations and under various circumstances. This approach is particularly concerned with the analyses of the ways of life pursued by those who acquire IHD compared to those of individuals who do not.

BIBLIOGRAPHY

ALBRINK, M. J., MEIGS, J. W., and MAN, E. B. 1961. Serum lipids, hypertension and coronary artery disease. *Am. J. Med.* 31:4.

ALBRINK, M. J., MEIGS, J. W., and GRANOFF, M. A. 1962. Weight gain and serum triglycerides in normal men. *New Engl. J. Med.* 266:484–89.

ANITSCHOW, N. 1914. Über die Atherosklerose der Aorta beim Kaninchen und über deren Entstehungsbedingungen. *Beitr. Pathol. Anat.* 59:306.

CHAPMAN, J. M., GOERKE, L. S., DIXON, W., LOVELAND, D. B., and PHILLIPS, E. 1957. The clinical status of a population group in Los Angeles under observation for two or three years. *Am. J. Public Health* 47:33–42.

DAWBER, T. R. and KANNEL, W. B. 1961. Susceptibility to coronary heart disease. Modern concepts of cardiovascular disease. New York: American Heart Association 30:671–76.

DAWBER, T. R., KANNEL, W. B., REVOTSKIE, N., and KAGAN, A. 1962. The epidemiology of coronary disease. The Framingham enquiry. *Proc. Roy. Soc. Med. (Sect. Epidemiol. Prev. Med.)* 55:265–71.

DORN, H. F. 1959. Tobacco consumption and mortality from cancer and other diseases. *Public Health Repts.* 74:581.

DOYLE, J. T., DAWBER, T. R., KANNEL, W. B., HASLIN, A. S., and KAHN, H. S. 1962. Cigarette smoking and coronary heart disease. *New Engl. J. Med.* 266:794–801.

ENOS, W. F., HOLMES, R. H., and BEYER, J. C. 1953. Coronary disease among United States soldiers killed in action in Korea. *J.A.M.A.* 152:1090–93.

FOX, S. M. and SKINNER, S. S. 1964. Physical activity and cardiovascular health. *Am. J. Cardiology* 14:731–46.

GERTLER, M. M. *et al.* 1954. *Coronary heart disease in young adults.* Cambridge, Mass.: Harvard University Press.

HERAPATH, C. E. K. and PERRY, C. B. 1930. The coronary arteries in a case of familial liability to sudden death. *Brit. Med. J.* 1:685.

HERRICK, J. B. 1912. Clinical features of sudden obstruction of the coronary artery. *J.A.M.A.* 59:2015.

———. 1919. Thrombosis of the coronary artery. *J.A.M.A.* 72:287.

KAHN, H. A. 1963. The relationship of reported coronary heart disease mortality to physical activity of work. *Am. J. Public Health* 53:1058–67.

LONGSTREET, T., KLEPETAR, E., KEYS, A., PARLIN, W., BLACKBURN, H., and PUCHNER, T. 1962. Death rates among physically active and sedentary employees of the railroad industry. *Am. J. Public Health* **52**:1697–1707.

MORRIS, J. N., HEADY, J. A., RAFFLER, P. A. B., ROBERTS, C. G., and PARKS, J. W. 1953. Coronary heart disease and physical activity work. I. Coronary heart disease in different occupations. II. Statement and testing of provisional hypothesis. *Lancet* **2**:1053, 1111.

MORRIS, J. N. 1961–62. Epidemiological aspects of ischaemic heart disease. *Yale J. Biol. Med.* **34**:359–69.

———. 1964. *Uses of epidemiology.* 2d ed, pp. 174–75. Edinburgh: E. & S. Livingstone.

PAUL, O., LEPPER, M. H., PHELAND, W. H., DUPERTUIS, G. W., MACMILLAN, A., McKEAN, H., and PARK, H. T. 1963. A longitudinal study of coronary heart disease. *Circulation* **28**:20–31.

PELL, S. and D'ALONZO, C. A. 1963. Acute myocardial infarction in a large industrial population. Report of a 6-year study of 1,356 cases. *J.A.M.A.* **185**:831–38.

RYLE, J. R. 1928. A note on John Hunter's cardiac infarct. *Lancet* **1**:332–34.

SHELDON, W. H. 1940. *The varieties of human physique.* New York: Harper & Bros.

SMOKING AND HEALTH. Report of the Advisory Committee to the Surgeon General of the Public Health Service. 1964. Public Health Service Publication No. 1103. Washington, D.C.: U.S. Government Printing Office.

THOMAS, C. B. and HIRSCHHORN, B. 1955. The familial occurrence of hypertension and coronary artery disease with observations concerning obesity and diabetes. *Ann. Int. Med.* **42**:90

WHITE, P D. 1957. The cardiologist enlists the epidemiologist. *Am. J. Public Health* **47**:1.

CHAPTER XX

Cancer

Any attempt to describe a subject as all-embracing as the epidemiology of cancer might be considered brash.[1] Actually it reminds me of attempts to describe the epidemiology of pneumonia, or even that mass of conditions which go under the name of infections. Indeed cancer, or malignant neoplasms, can be so extremely variegated in their structure or behavior that it is hard to characterize them as belonging to a single group. Possibly the only features that human cancers have in common are (*a*) the unbridled manner in which the cells tend to grow (and even this may be an artificial or arbitrary measure); and (*b*) malignant neoplasm usually causes the eventual death of the afflicted patient, if the tumor has progressed beyond that stage when it can be successfully extirpated. And yet in spite of the gloomy prognosis under which this chapter starts out, it is not a complete waste of time to consider the numerous and heterogeneous kinds of lesions together, and to review the variety of circumstances under which some of them arise. At least such an exercise has the virtue of getting one adjusted to think along those lines peculiar to the cancer field. Of course, one could take up certain individual anatomical types of cancer one by one—lung, stomach, prostate, and so forth—but I shall have to forego any such an attempt for a variety of reasons, particularly if this book is to be kept at all within bounds.

First let us look at the matter of nosology, that is, the system of nomenclature and classification under which cancers have been

---

[1] Much of this chapter has been taken from an unpublished article entitled "The Epidemiological Approach to Cancer Research," written by this author in 1961 at the request of the American Cancer Society.

identified for well over 100 years, a system that has followed the time-honored principle of identifying anatomically the organ from whence the type of cancer cell arose, and later whether they were derived from epithelial, connective tissue or other types of cells. This system has proved useful in practical matters such as pathological and surgical diagnosis, although perhaps less so in matters of taxonomy. Nevertheless elements of etiology and various types of carcinogens of a physical or chemical nature have begun to be recognized with growing frequency. More recently, viruses as possible etiologic agents have come on the scene. Thus it has begun to be conceivable to some that a system of identification and classification comparable to that long in use for infections might eventually be applied to cancers. This would mean rewriting the old anatomical classification into one with new terms by taking on, when it could, etiologic considerations as well as anatomic ones. But Clemmesen (1965) has sounded a note of warning about classifying neoplasms prematurely on the basis of their etiology, largely because of incomplete knowledge about their causes as well as the multiplicity and variability of these causes. He says: "Under these circumstances the mere demonstration of one or other carcinogen in some environment will in no way correspond to the demonstration of bacteria or viruses in infection epidemiology, nor will the application of Koch's criteria be permissible." For instance, although cancers that develop as a result of the same occupational exposure are similar, some carcinogens of viral origin are inclined to cause different histologic structures and invade different organs.

So the anatomical system long in use is not ready to be changed yet, and, in fact, that change would seem to be a long way off. We are still in a position comparable to one occupied one hundred years ago by those medical scientists of the pre-Pasteurian era, who, although eager to learn the cause of infections knew practically nothing about bacteria.

HISTORY

Perhaps the earliest, and certainly the most frequently quoted, early observation on an occupational carcinogen came from

Percival Pott of London, who described in 1775, scrotal tumors prone to occur in chimney sweeps, who when young had been assigned to this unsavory trade—a trade fortunately disappearing today. This was an isolated observation and the concept of the epidemiology of neoplasms can hardly have been said to have begun until 100 years later. Indeed, most of the individual efforts made along these lines from about 1870 until about 1920 were the speculations of geographically minded pathologists, not of trained epidemiologists—for there were few of the latter in existence. Although Rous had reported on his sarcoma virus in chickens as early as 1911, pathologists (and perhaps surgeons also) in the late nineteenth and early twentieth centuries, who were pioneers in cancer research, were understandably, primarily interested in how to identify individual tumors, in what methods were useful in the clinical diagnosis of various kinds of tumors, and in how these tumors behaved. Such activities were soon followed by work in the laboratory on experimental cancer, on genetics, carcinogens, endocrines, and the transplantation of tumors.[2]

Epidemiological thinking about cancer may be said to have begun when Rigoni Stern (quoted by Clemmesen, 1965) collected cancer mortality statistics for the city of Verona beginning in 1842; followed by Tanchou who reported on causes of death in Paris in 1843. In the latter half of the nineteenth century, others reviewed the occurrence of cancer from widely scattered places, including A. Haviland (1870) who pointed out that in England the geographical distribution of cancer was irregular, a phenomenon demonstrable even within the limits of one small country. But the global aspect of the situation was taken up by August Hirsch in the second edition of his famous *Handbook of Geographical and Historical Pathology* (1886) who said: "Defective as these conclusions are for the whole geographical distribution of cancer, they serve at least to make certain that

[2] For a review of this period in cancer research, see: Charles Oberling, *The Riddle of Cancer*, translated by W. H. Woglum (New Haven, Yale University Press, 1944); or Isaac Berenblum, *Man against Cancer, The Story of Cancer Research* (Baltimore, John Hopkins Press, 1952).

climatic influences do not affect the frequency of the disease." Hoffman's book dealing with differential mortality rates and the geographical pathology of cancer throughout the world did not appear until 1915. Next came large-scale urban studies, several of them carried out by the U.S. Public Health Service. During this period and before, isolated observations and claims had been made about the high prevalence of certain kinds of malignant tumors in betel-nut chewers, and the low prevalence in other primitive populations such as Navaho Indians or Eskimos. Then came a more concerted search for environmental influences, occupations, and ways of living that might be responsible for these gradients. The alertness of Martland *et al.* (1925) who observed the sarcomata that occurred among those whose occupation was to paint watch dials with radioactive substances is a special and unique case in point. His was the first recognition of malignancy induced by ingested radioactive substances. He also pointed out ways to control the lesion.

It was not long, however, before it became abundantly apparent that it was not easy to measure the prevalence of cancer in a given population by the usual available means. Problems of diagnosis, particularly in developing countries, are notoriously difficult. Furthermore, the age structure of a population, as illustrated in Fig. 16, and its age-specific death rate should be known before much interpretation can be attempted. Most cases and most deaths from cancer occur after middle age, at a time of life when there is more competition from various causes of death than in young adult life (see Fig. 39). Thus the prevalence of cancer will be influenced to a marked degree not only by the availability of old people but by the relative prevalence of other "diseases of old age." Take for instance the incredibly young age at which the average Eskimo dies, from accidents, epidemics, and so on. How can he be expected to live to acquire the cancers from which most North American urban populations suffer?

It is perhaps superfluous to add that in the pursuit of various epidemiological techniques it is necessary to assemble large numbers of the population at risk if rates of any particular variety of cancer are to be considered significant or even comparable to others. In this country, a milestone was passed in the implementation of these techniques with the publication of the review by Dorn and Cutler (1958) dealing with *Morbidity of Cancer in the United States.*

That cancer was and is an important cause of death in civilized countries is generally recognized. But that in the United States it

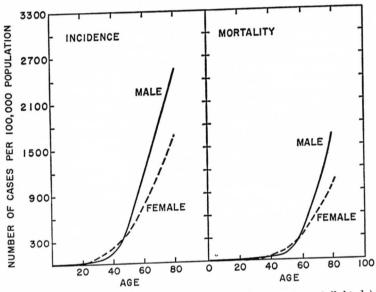

FIG. 39. Cancer age-specific incidence and mortality rates (all kinds) listed by sex, New York State excluding New York City, 1958–60. (Data from Shimkin, M. B., 1964. Science and cancer. Public Health Service Publication No. 1162, p. 12.)

now ranks number two as a cause of death comes as a surprise. This prominence of cancer is true for Canada, most of Europe, Australia and New Zealand and apparently for the U.S.S.R. What brought this situation about among the most highly developed countries in the world? Partial explanations can be found in the improved manner in which various types of cancer are reported; in the conquest of infectious diseases; in ways that have been instrumental in prolonging life expectancy, and in an increase in industrialized civilizations that have brought man in closer contact with carcinogens. Much of this high rate for cancer is due, of course, to unknown causes.

To obtain proper measurements of the prevalence, incidence, or death rates of a disease is the first task of the epidemiologist. This is not easily accomplished with cancer. To offset difficulties there has been a growing effort to establish and maintain tumor registries in various places. These have sometimes proved of immense local value, as well as being of use for comparing one population with another. The Connecticut Tumor Registry, started shortly after World War II, when Connecticut's population was not much over 2,000,000, was a pioneer effort in the United States. Such registries have been set up in a number of states in the United States, and also in several countries—Norway, Denmark, Sweden, and England. Clemmesen's (1965) registry from 1943 to 1957 in Denmark is particularly noteworthy.

Obviously the size of the population from which the registry is drawn will influence its efficiency. This size should be sufficiently large to yield data adequate for analyses and should at the same time be small enough to enable an intimate study of the situation. It is generally estimated that a population of about 4,000,000 is a valuable size. At the same time it is assumed that a population worthy of having a registry is one provided with adequate medical and health facilities so that most cases of neoplasms can be properly diagnosed and handled, and the diagnoses adequately recorded and coded. A heartening number of observations have resulted from these tumor registries. In several instances leads have emerged that have stimulated new studies, both retrospective and prospective, a good many of which are now in progress.

Geographic Distribution

Not the least of the functions of tumor registries and other local surveys on the epidemiology of cancer has been to provide a satisfactory statistical basis for making comparisons between different places and populations—an approach commonly referred to as the geographical pathology of cancer. This has been no easy task. Thus a conference on Geographical Pathology and Demography of Cancer, held in Oxford in 1950, brought forth a lively discussion between pathologists and epidemiologists on how to map areas of greater or lesser incidence and how to interpret the results—for there seemed to be profound differences in points of view between pathologists and statisticians. At that time statistical epidemiology was not only on the rise (Top 1952) but an established science; and it had become apparent that if standard or consistent results were to be obtained, there would have to be adherence to certain epidemiologic techniques. Such techniques have now been summarized in a useful booklet edited by Doll (1959).

Subsequently, numbers of pathologists have been quick to adopt epidemiological methods and have become excellent epidemiologists both in the field of cancer and elsewhere; for after all, pathology is hardly limited to the study of the morphology of tumors. It embraces the nature and causes of disease and should be approached by any legitimate method that the pathologist sees fit to use—even epidemiological techniques.

In all areas, regardless of race or color, the inhabitants develop cancer of one type or another. The relative frequency of different types of cancer differ significantly in various places, but, as already mentioned, this is a question of degree. Thus in the United States and many European countries the most common forms of cancer among women are those of the breast, uterus, and large intestine; among men, the lung, prostate, and large intestine rank highest as causes of death (Segi, 1960). These values sometimes change. For instance, cancer of the stomach has decreased in the United States. It is now seen most frequently in cold climates in the lower socioeconomic levels, notably among people of Iceland, Scandinavia, Russia, and Japan. In contrast are lower rates of breast cancer in Japan and of uterine cervical cancer in Israel, and in Jewish women of other countries. Compare for instance what one would find in a series of examinations of the alimentary tracts of adult Japanese and adult Americans. Cancers of the stomach would be six times as likely to occur in the Japanese as in the American but cancers of the colon would be nearly five times as likely to occur in the Americans as in the Japanese.

These international comparisons are more meaningful, of course, when based on data from countries where adequate and standard cancer registration systems exist and when proper age adjustments of the death rates have been made. Some of the differences are explainable on ethnic as well as other grounds. For instance, skin cancer ranks high among fair-skinned males, although this is not apparent in mortality statistics because most patients with skin cancer are successfully treated. Differing average annual death rate for whites and nonwhites from leukemia in the first five years of life is also a case in point (Slocumb and MacMahon 1963).

Of special interest has been the continent of Africa. Attention has been called to the prevalence of certain types of cancer in a huge district which covers most of the southern portion of the African continent (Higginson and Oettle 1960). Here cancer of the esophagus has been noted with special frequency. Another more limited area is in Mozambique, where cancer of the liver is common. Another African tumor that has attracted considerable attention is a lymphosarcoma, or perhaps leukosarcoma, often of the jaw or face (Burkitt's tumor) and most frequently seen in children. It has been found in East Africa, particularly in Kenya and Uganda, and is said to be uncommon elsewhere. A good reason for its notoriety is that its distribution has been said to follow water courses and this has suggested the possibility of its being mosquito-borne. Dalldorf (1962) has suggested that it is a variety of juvenile lymphatic leukemia that for some strange reason assumes the guise of leukosarcoma in this part of the African continent. Vigorous efforts are being made to see if it is transmissible to primates.

GEOGRAPHICAL LEADS

Having assembled a certain amount of data on the differential prevalence of varieties of cancer in given places, the epidemiologist's task, like that of the pathologist, has just begun. His next step is a search for measurable factors that can account for these differing rates. Local pollution of the atmosphere, local occupations and industries, diet, habits, and customs whether religious or political should all come in for their share of scrutiny. It is extremely difficult to separate racial predilections from local customs and environmental conditions, and indeed it would seem hardly worthwhile to make great efforts to differentiate them. The important thing is whether a measurable factor, such as smoking an excess of cigarettes and lung cancer, exists.

One important project is that being devised by investigators who have hit upon the ingenious idea of studying at least three populations of Japanese, each living in a different environment—in Japan, in Hawaii, and in California. To some extent each of these populations retain common customs, but they are exposed to different types of terrain, probably to different diets, and to a variety of other influences that may or may not affect the rates at which cancers of one sort or another could develop.

Variegated Causes

When it comes to assigning a definite cause or even a single item that can be designated as a cause of cancer, one soon finds oneself in a quandry. For instance, although genetic influences have long been suspected it is but a few years since attention was first called to the increased rate of leukemia amongst those afflicted with mongolism; and Wilms tumor is more likely to occur in association with congenital anomalies of the genital tract. There are other isolated examples but the question of a true hereditary or racial predisposition to cancer remains controversial. Clemmesen (1965) has maintained that none of the numerous genetic studies has succeeded in demonstrating a general hereditary disposition to human cancer as a whole.

Furthermore, the list of carcinogetic agents to which man is susceptible grows annually in length and variety. Chemicals, many of them tars and dyes, head the list. We know that exposure to cigarette smoke accounts for most of the present incidence of lung cancer; also it may be produced by chromate ore and mustard gas processing.[3] Asbestos production and exposure to nickel refining processes can be responsible for cancer of the nasal sinuses. Also, we know that some aromatic amines and related compounds produce cancer of the urinary bladder. In fact, although Hueper (1954) assembled an extensive list of industrial carcinogens and the occupations known to be hazardous on their account, more have been discovered since. To mention a few of those to which one is exposed in daily life, we know that carcinoma of the skin can be induced by natural ultraviolet radiation as well as by a great number of chemicals. Ionizing radiation can produce leukemia and cancer in other organs as a result of both short and prolonged exposures; and indeed a great variety of agents can be carcinogenetic on occasion: such as thermal burns, air pollutants, and on the endogenous side, hormones, to mention only a few. It is an arresting list for a disease whose cause is so often said to be unknown.

Although it may not yet apply to man, the recent resurgence of interest in viruses as possible carcinogenetic agents, which began in the 1930's, has captured the imagination of many. In various animal species there are now at least a dozen cancers that are of established viral etiology. The discovery by Shope of the Rockefeller Institute in 1933, who succeeded in passing benign papillomata from wild rabbits to domestic rabbits and showed that in the latter species, these papillomata assumed the characteristic of malignant growths, was a case in point. The observation by Bittner of the Jackson Memorial Laboratory of Bar Harbor in 1937 that some carcinogenetic agent was transmissible in the mother's milk of mice to the offspring was another important landmark. Several other tumor-producing viral agents were soon brought to light, although up to the present time no human cancer has been shown to be due to a virus. And yet experience with animal viruses is now so extensive that it is unlikely that a human example may not soon be uncovered. Why is it so difficult

[3] The Japanese mustard gas factory that was discovered to be the source of cancer of the lung and respiratory tract among the employees in the early 1950's is a case in point.

to isolate viruses from tumors? Does the crux of this virus-host relationship lie mainly within the host who requires a special type of conditioning to make him susceptible? These problems remain to be solved.

One is brought to the conclusions that the human race (and perhaps animals) are beset with many carcinogenetic agents and that man becomes particularly vulnerable after age 50. These agents alone or in combination seem ready to make their presence felt at the appropriate time of life. Of this consideration we should be reminded by a glance at Fig. 39, and a restatement of Loeb's (1945) law: "The organism, its constituent parts, and their associated cancers each has its own characteristic time curve." In other words, conditioning of the soil, either purely by age or by factors within the climate in which one lives, may play a greater role in the cancer process than has been credited to it.

It may well be that the optimum age span is not merely a reflection of aging but of a long incubation period or of long exposure to a carcinogen. For instance, one has to be exposed to aniline dyes for some time before such chemicals become a grave threat in producing bladder carcinomata. Or one has to have used cigarettes in excess of twenty years or more before the chances of acquiring carcinomata of the lung are enhanced.

A legitimate question might be raised over this matter of age and aging and its relation to the cancer process. This would be whether all cancers behave true to form, which is certainly not the case. There are sarcomata of the bones of the limbs, for instance, that occur in individuals of both sexes who are relatively young, whereas if one considers the bones other than those of the limbs, the neoplastic lesion is apt to occur in older people, and there is a distinct gradient between male and female. We seem to have two clinical pictures based on two anatomical locations involving the same type of tissue. And several tumors located in a similar organ can be differentiated on the basis of the cell types that determine their individuality. Thus testicular teratomata tend to arise in relatively young people, whereas seminomas occur in older age groups. Many other tumors have an optimum age span, several occurring in the very young such as the acute leukemias of infancy, where exposure to radiation in utero may have influenced the process unfavorably (Stewart 1961, MacMahon 1962).

ENVIRONMENTAL INFLUENCES

Rather than try to track down individual carcinogenic agents at this point, it may be worthwhile for the cancer epidemiologist to review ways of living that seem to promote various types of cancer. For instance, those ways of urban life, which seem to be perfectly normal to us now, may eventually be as unacceptable as were those of seventeenth and eighteenth century urban Europe. The smoking of tobacco, particularly in the form of cigarettes, apparently accounts for a major proportion of the increases in lung cancers during the past 20 years. It has been difficult to persuade the smoking public in America, however, that there is sufficient reason for it to change its smoking habits and give up cigarettes. Nevertheless such associations call for a re-estimate of modern ways of living. A valuable study along these lines is now being carried out among a group of Seventh Day Adventists who happen to be living in Los Angeles, California. The habits of the sect are guided by certain religious laws or principles and in this respect these individuals represent persons with specific ways of living. These include restriction of diets, in some instances to a vegetarian regime, the avoidance of alcohol and tobacco, and a variety of other features subject to analyses.

RESIDENTIAL CONDITIONS

In spite of fast-diminishing differences between city and country life in general, city dwellers have up to three times more lung cancer than rural inhabitants, a difference not thought to be accounted for by differences in smoking habits. A great proportion of this gradient is thought to be due to air pollution caused by industrial wastes, automobile exhausts, and household sources. In the United States, Drinker (1961) is more cautious, however, in his statement that a relationship has not been found between carcinogens in cigarette smoke and those in polluted city air. In Denmark and England, the urban mortality rates are higher for all cancers, in fact 15 to 40 per cent higher than those of rural residents.

SOCIOECONOMIC STATUS

There seems to be a relationship between socioeconomic status and cancer incidence. Clemmesen and Nielsen in Copenhagen (1951) and Stocks (1947) in England have shown that certain trends exist in these countries; and Cohart and Muller (1955) have reported similar findings which concern cancer of the gastro-intestinal tract in New Haven, Connecticut. Dorn and Cutler (1958) summarized these findings with the statement that a fairly regular inverse gradient of cancer incidence and socio-economic class was observed for all forms of cancer among white males and among non-white males and females. Among white females, the incidence of cancer was 14 per cent above average in the lower classes but occurred with equal frequency in the four other income classes; on the other hand, cancer of the breast occurred somewhat more frequently in the higher income classes.

Personal habits and attributes. Diets deficient in proteins and vitamins may be associated with cancer of the oral cavity, pharynx, and esophagus. Diet is also probably involved in cancer of the liver, stomach, and other digestive organs. Smoking and cancer of the lung will be taken up in chapter 21. The frequency of breast cancer is higher among nulliparous women than multiparous women. Conversely, cancer of the uterine cervix occurs oftener among women who have experienced an active sexual and reproductive life. Cancer of the penis is rarely seen among circumcised males.

IONIZING RADIATION

Ionizing radiation has been mentioned already in connection with occupational cancer and with therapeutic and diagnostic radiation (Lindell and Dobson 1961). That leukemia can be produced in man by the kind of ionizing radiation produced by atomic bombs is now established. The literature has been summarized by Hollingsworth (1960). Evidence of the leukemogenic effect of this exposure is strongly supported by the observation that the incidence of leukemia was highest in those who received the heaviest exposure. The existence of a relationship between such exposure to the bombs and other kinds of cancer is not so clear.

GENERAL THEORIES

This chapter is being rapidly reduced to a long list of factors, some closely related, others distantly related, that seem to have something to do with the cancer-inducing process. But the crux of the problem nevertheless—the over-all processes by which cancer is produced—remains unanswered. We come instead to an evaluation of various theories that deal with the pathogenesis of cancer. Our analysis of these is given so as to create certain focal points which may serve as hooks on which the epidemiologist can hang his ideas.

In general, it would seem unlikely, to the author at least, that one fundamental process is responsible for all cancers. Nevertheless a reasonable and broad premise might be that malignancy arises from the same three major influences, mentioned before in this book in an agricultural simile: the seed, the soil, and the climate. Possibly the soil and the climate should receive most attention in the cancerous process.

Among those theories about cancer that have long been considered a few stand out: (1) there is an innate (embryonal or genetic) general cellular tendency to neoplastic growth that occurs autonomously in certain individuals or may be brought about as a result of minor outside influences or humoral factors; (2) the major influence is a direct effect of certain physical or chemical carcinogens, including radiation, exerted upon cells, which in turn depends on the capacity of the cell to respond; (3) the normal cell is invaded presumably by a virus or viruses or other parasitic agents.[4]

[4] These and other theories have been variously proposed by many authors and the literature of the past generation contains literally volumes devoted to their consideration. Oberling (1944) deals with this question by giving three major hypotheses: the irritative, the embryonal, and the microbic parasite. If compared to our three theories given above, these represent a slight shift in order to: 2, 1, and 3.

Granted that these three theories might be taken up in order, as long as there is good reason to believe that host susceptibility is a pre-eminent factor in the induction of cancer, it may be of some advantage to begin our discussion with a consideration of the "soil" or host. Thus host cells might be more capable of yielding a neoplastic response when conditioned by the number of chromosomes within cells, an excess or a lack of hormones, or circumstances associated with advancing age (Fig. 39). The reasoning harks back to our theory number 1. In support of its adherents, Starr (1960) has called attention to the rather constant proportion with which a small fraction of the population develops fatal cancer in many different countries with vastly differing populations. He says:

Despite the manifold sources from which the cancerous subpopulations may be recruited, it is a remarkable fact that the cancer mortality in any population is predictable, fairly constant, and varies within narrow limits. . . . Deaths from cancer vary between 0.03 and 0.3 per cent, the higher rates being encountered where superior public health services prevail.

To reconcile this with any theory one must assume that tumor viruses and the various carcinogens, known or unknown, must be as universal or endemic as are pneumococci or streptococci in their global distribution.

Perhaps this is mindful of Cramer's (1942) law propagated about twenty-five years ago; that the total mortality rate for cancer of all kinds in women in England, Holland, Switzerland, and Japan was approximately the same, although the distribution of the sites of these cancers varied considerably. Nevertheless, Cramer's law seems to have gone out of fashion. It is clear it would not hold for men, considering the increase in bronchial carcinoma particularly among urban males in Western countries.

Theory 2 alleges that the seed may be dominant. Obviously various kinds of agents cause neoplasms, but in the absence of actual experimental tests on humans of all ages under a wide variety of conditions, one may still have to wait a long time before there is a proper understanding of the nature of the biologic equilibrium between seed and soil. Some carcinogens conceivably can cause neoplasms in man at almost any age, others may require special circumstances.

As for theory number 3, it may be that the seed is really dominant here. No one can venture far in his explanations of cancer etiology without being confronted with the question of the parasitic etiology in general, and a virus etiology in particular for some cancers. The matter has been the subject of a number of recent studies, notably one by a W.H.O. Study Group (1965). But although one is prone to seek a single cause for cancer, it is not reasonable to restrict carcinogenic stimuli to any one class of agents, viruses or otherwise.

But to return to a review of what has proved to be a multiplicity of theories about cancer, at least one can be mentioned that primarily concerns the precancerous cell. It stems from new observations and new knowledge that have arisen from work on passage cell lines in tissue culture in the past five or ten years. Thus it has been observed that explanted normal human cells, when cultivated serially, undergo alteration that enables them to multiply autonomously, and to all intents and purposes indefinitely, under well-defined conditions. These cells sometimes undergo malignant change in this artificial environment. Such a concept prompts the idea that a like mutation of one cell in many millions could conceivably occur naturally in various parts of the body and at all times of life. But this would not be dangerous as long as the protective mechanisms with which the body is normally endowed, could hold the mutated cells in check. But the theory would also assume that, as a general phenomenon in man these hypothetical protective mechanisms, controlling the new growth of mutating cells, might wear out with advancing age. This process would be a manifestation of one of many aging processes, such as the decline of non-specific antibodies. This is probably an oversimplification of what is a very complex process, but in any event, comparative studies of a number of immune mechanisms including non-specific antibody titers in normal old people and in cancerous old people deserve study—and, indeed, such studies have been started.

One could go on speculating at some length about such theories, but this is not the function of this chapter. The function is, rather, to point out that the epidemiologist is in a key position to explore many new leads and areas of cancer research.

Although it is not the purpose of this book to recommend or even suggest particular lines of research, I have drawn from a recent W.H.O. report (*Viruses and Cancer* 1965) a number of useful observations about the epidemiological approach. In stressing the multiplicity of factors involved, this report shows that such epidemiological studies of cancer require the collection of data from numerous sources—medical, veterinary, biological, social, and others—emphasizing how the assistance of local cancer registration centers can help in detecting and evaluating clusters of cases. Certainly it is important that these clusters (or their absence) be observed over wide areas.

Another factor is a thorough appreciation of the long latent period between exposure of a carcinogen and the development of the lesion. The report points out that some of the difficulties may be lessened by studying childhood cancers and by including the possible role of viruses in the malignant neoplasms of the hemapoetic and reticular systems.

It mentions furthermore, that although there is no reason to suspect transmission of animal cancer viruses to man, the possibility that this has occurred or can occur cannot be ignored. At least we can gain insight into cancer processes by observation of the natural history of spontaneous cancer in animals. There is evidence to suggest, for instance, that bovine lymphosarcoma, cat leukemia, and pulmonary adenomatosis of sheep are communicable within the respective animal species. Epizootical studies should therefore be extended.

CONCLUSION

This is only the briefest epitome of a little understood subject, and it has suffered from attempts at simplification and has other shortcomings. It may serve, however, as an introduction for anyone contemplating a study of the clinical epidemiology of certain forms of cancer.

BIBLIOGRAPHY

BERENBLUM, I. 1952. *Man against cancer, the story of cancer research.* Baltimore: Johns Hopkins Press.

CLEMMESEN, J. and NIELSEN, A. 1951. The social distribution of cancer in Copenhagen in 1943–1947. *Brit. J. Cancer* **5**:159–71.

CLEMMESEN, J. 1965 a. *Statistical studies in the aetiology of malignant neoplasms, I. Review and results.* Copenhagen: Munksgaard.

———. 1965 b. *Statistical studies in the aetiology of malignant neoplasms, II. Basic tables, Denmark 1943–57.* Copenhagen: Munksgaard.

COHART, E. M. and MULLER, C.: 1955. Socioeconomic distribution of cancer of the gastro-intestinal tract in New Haven. *Cancer* **8**:378–88.

CRAMER, W. O. 1942. The origin of cancer in man. *J.A.M.A.* **119**:309–16.

DORN, H. F. and CUTLER, S. J. 1958. Morbidity from cancer in the United States. Public Health Monographs No. 56, pp. 207. Washington, D.C.: U.S. Government Printing Office.

DALLDORF, G. 1962. Lymphomas of African children with different forms of environmental influences *J.A.M.A.* **181**:1026–28.

DOLL, R. (ed.). 1959. *Methods of geographical pathology.* Springfield, Ill.: Charles C Thomas.

DRINKER, P. 1961. Air pollution. *New Engl. J. Med.* **264**:754–59.

HAVILAND, A. 1870. Geographical distribution of diseases in England and Wales. II. Cancer. *Brit. Med. J.* **2**:573–75.

HIGGINSON, J. and OETTLE, A. G. 1960. Cancer incidence in the Bantu and "Cape Colored" races of South Africa: report of a cancer survey in the Transvaal (1953–55) *J. Nat. Cancer Inst.* **24**:589–671.

HIRSCH, A. 1886. *Handbook of geographical and historical pathology.* Translated from the 2d ed. by C. C. CREIGHTON. III, 502–9. London: New Sydenham Society.

HOFFMAN, F. L. 1915. *The mortality from cancer throughout the world.* Newark, N.J.: Prudential Press.

HOLLINGSWORTH, J. W. 1960. Delayed radiation effects in survivors of atomic bombings. *New Engl. J. Med.* **263**:481–87.

HUEPER, W. C. 1954. Recent developments in environmental cancer. *Arch. Path.* **58**:360–99; 475–523; 645–82.

LINDELL, B. and DOBSON, R. L. 1961. Ionizing radiation and health. Public Health Papers No. 6. Geneva: World Health Organization.

LOEB, L. 1945. Cancer and the process of ageing. In *Biological Symposia* Vol. 11, ed. R. A. MOORE, pp. 197–216. Lancaster, Pa.; Jacques Cattell Press.

MacMahon, B. 1962. Prenatal exposure and childhood cancer. *J. Nat. Cancer Inst.* **28**:1173–91.

MacMahon, B. and Levy, M. A. 1964. Prenatal origin of childhood leukemia. Evidence from twins. *New Engl. J. Med.* **270**:1082–85.

Martland, H. S., Condon, P., and Knef, J. P. 1925. Unrecognized dangers in use and handling of radioactive substances; with especial reference to storage of insoluble products of radium and mesothorium in the reticulo-endothelial system. *J.A.M.A.* **85**:1769–76.

Oberling, C. 1944. The riddle of cancer. Translated by W. H. Woglom, pp. 17–37. New Haven; Yale University Press.

Segi, M. 1960. *Cancer mortality for selected sites in 24 countries (1950–1957).* Sendai, Japan: Tohoku University School of Medicine.

Shimkin, M. B. 1964. Science and cancer. Public Health Service Report No. 1162. Washington, D.C.: Department of Health, Education, and Welfare.

Starr, K. W. 1960. Bilogical equilibria in human cancer. *Nature* **186**:1006–10.

Stewart, A. 1961. Aetiology of childhood malignancies. Congenitally determined leukemias. *Brit. Med. J.* **1**:542–60.

Stocks, P. 1947. Regional and local differences in cancer death rates. Studies on Medical and Population Subjects, No. 1. London: His Majesty's Stationery Office.

Top, F. M. (ed.). 1952. *History of American epidemiology.* St. Louis: C. V. Mosby Co.

Viruses and cancer. 1965. W.H.O. Technical Report Series, No. 295. Geneva.

CHAPTER XXI

Smoking and Carcinoma of the Lung

Carcinoma of the lung and its relationship to excessive cigarette smoking has been chosen for review for two particular reasons: first, because it has been brought to light mainly as an example of brilliant epidemiological detective work; and second, because it has been resisted, with extraordinary stubborness, by many good medical scientists who will not accept the evidence and will not even listen to any part of it. Others who do not like the idea have been unwilling to accept the evidence either as unconvincing or that they would prefer to wait for a while. Some scientists have resisted accepting the evidence on cigarette smoking and lung cancer because they have not been willing to accept practically any conclusion based on statistical epidemiological data, particularly when the time-honored sciences of pathology, histology, and genetics have not pointed to any such conclusions in the past. Perhaps suspicion or distrust of evidence produced by purely statistical methods has been so deeply inbred that it is impossible to supplant it. Others have maintained that the statistical methods used were inadequate and failed to produce crucial evidence.

It should be mentioned first of all that unless one is willing to accept statistical evidence to document the association between excessive cigarette smoking and lung cancer, there is little use in going further with this chapter. True, we have considered statistical methods and epidemiological evidence throughout the entire book, but it becomes particularly pertinent in this chapter (Weaver 1960). It was not, for instance, until biostatisticians assembled enough data on enough individuals who smoked cigarettes heavily in contrast to those who did not that this information came to light. Fortunately, smoking stood out as the prominent factor in these statistical investigations and was not clouded by other multiple causes. Clinical, pathological, and experimental bits of evidence have been invoked but not nearly on such a large scale.

The first question is, of course, whether an association between excessive cigarette smoking and lung cancer actually exists. If this premise is accepted, the next question is whether this association has causal significance. Such questions have been considered in the report of the Advisory Committee to the Surgeon General of the U.S. Public Health Service entitled *Smoking and Health* (1964). Five points are stressed in this association: its consistency, strength, specificity, temporal relationship, and coherence. These points will not be taken up one by one but some attention will be paid to each.

It is possible that the remarks regarding the relationship of excessive cigarette smoking to lung cancer may sound too didactic. Some of the five points or criteria mentioned in the Surgeon General's report may sound as if I have treated them as being completely settled rather than as assumptions. Indeed, all is not settled with regard to this relationship, but according to my opinion and that of many others the evidence so far is convincing.

A word about method may be in order here. The main epidemiologic ways for digging out evidence of this kind when large numbers are necessary to make one's point, are retrospective and prospective surveys. The retrospective approach usually starts with a series of cases and proceeds to determine whether a given association of a given hypothesis is fulfilled by any or a number of these cases. It matches then, age for age, and in other fashions, an equal or greater number of controls drawn from the local population or other groups; and an association is sought in an effort to determine what degree of expected correlation would be found in a general population. To get a good comparison one should have as large a number of cases and controls as one can conveniently handle. Furthermore, the sources of bias may be endless. The prospective method calls for the testing of an association or hypothesis in a series of individuals who have not yet acquired the disease in question. One chooses not a series of cases but a population, perhaps one divided into cohorts. The population is observed for a given number of years or at least until enough data is accumulated to make the survey meaningful.

Within the last century the use of cigarettes has become as commonplace as that of bread and milk. To challenge their use is to criticize the habits of tens of millions of Americans, as well as one of the nation's major industries. In the last fifty years the consumption of cigarettes has gone up tremendously, whereas cigar and pipe smoking has declined. A glance at Fig. 40 will

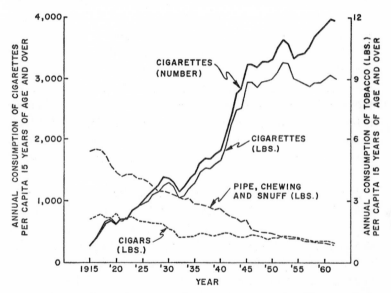

Fig. 40. Trends in tobacco use. Consumption per capita, 15 years of age and over. United States, 1915–62. (Data from *Cigarette Smoking and Health*. A Review of studies by the California State Department of Health, California State Board of Health, 1963.)

show some of these relationships and also will explain in part why the U.S. Surgeon General's Committee got such a cool response from its report when it appeared in January, 1964, and during subsequent months.

HISTORICAL NOTE

Perhaps before pursuing this critical attitude further we should turn our attention to the history of the discovery of the association between lung cancer and smoking, and to the wealth of evidence that has appeared in the past decade, so that the reader may decide how convincing this evidence has been. At first the evidence was vague but arresting, beginning arbitrarily with Lombard and Doering's observations in Massachusetts (1928). Later Raymond Pearl (1938) had some things to say about it that should not be forgotten. When in 1950 a famous surgeon, Evarts Graham, began reporting a preponderance of heavy smokers among his large series lung cancer cases, people began to take notice but not many considered the association seriously. Subsequently, during the 1950's and 1960's, E. L. Wynder (1961) has been a diligent worker in this vineyard.

In the first third of the twentieth century, physicians and pathologists began to notice what seemed to be a real increase in the number of cases of lung cancer, far transcending any other sudden increase in other types of cancer. I well remember my sojourn in the 1920's as a pathologist at the Pennsylvania Hospital in Philadelphia, where the autopsy service had been established at the turn of the century under Simon Flexner and later maintained by Warfield Longcope. Such men would not have missed many cases of lung cancer had it been common in their time (1898–1909), and the annals of that hospital reveal it decidedly was not. Carefully kept record books testify to the rarity of lung cancer. In the 1920's bronchiogenic carcinoma had become more common, and was more common still in the 1930's, to which the report of Bauer testifies (1933). Furthermore, it was almost entirely restricted to the male sex. This experience was by no means unique for this hospital; in fact it was almost universal throughout the United States for any general hospital. It was the beginning of an upsurge in which far more cases were recorded in the next two decades.

By 1950, public health authorities as well as pathologists had become concerned over this noticeable increase in lung cancer—

an increase that has continued to the present time. Various reasons were presented: the great increase in the consumption of cigarettes (Fig. 39), and the increase in air pollution from automobile exhausts and from industrial fumes. The air-pollution hypothesis seemed plausible since lung cancer death rates were reported to be higher in urban than in rural surroundings. In the meantime biostatisticians (Doll and Hill 1950) had brought their attention to this problem in a series of studies in which 20 London hospitals joined. They actually took the problem under their wings so to speak. Indeed, it is hard to see how a definitive answer could have been reached without recourse to a method in which adequate numbers of individuals are considered and adequate numbers of cases of lung cancer are assembled.

One can single out for review a few of the key pioneer studies; prominent among them was the work of Richard Doll and Bradford Hill in England (1956), and Hammond and Horn in the United States (1958). The former group were distinctly blazing the trail, their initial inquiries being sent out in 1951. A preliminary report was made in 1954 and a second report by Doll and Hill appeared in 1956. In 1951, these authors had dispatched over 40,000 questionnaires to men and women members of the medical profession in the United Kingdom and were able to amass information about the smoking habits of these physicians at that time. These physicians were classified as: non-smokers and smokers (or ex-smokers), the latter being divided into three main groups according to the amount of tobacco they smoked. The mortality of each group was recorded nearly four and a half years later (Doll and Hill 1956) from lung cancer and other causes. Their estimate of mortality in relation to the amount smoked at different ages above 35, appears in Table 11.

In the United States, Hammond and Horn (1958) of the American Cancer Society conducted a large scale enquiry from 1952 to 1955 covering the records of 187,783 men from 50 to 69 years of age. Their objectives were to relate smoking habits to the total death rates and to the deaths from lung cancer and a few other diagnoses. Perhaps the most significant finding was concerned with smoking habits and bronchiogenic carcinoma (exclusive of adenocarcinoma) (see Fig. 41). Here the data are shown and the association would seem to be extremely high. On the other hand, this team also found an important association between cigarette smoking and total death rate from various causes, in which coronary disease accounted for 51.1 per cent of the ex-

TABLE 11

AGE-SPECIFIC MORTALITY FROM LUNG CANCER IN
BRITISH PHYSICIANS; ANNUAL RATES PER 1,000 MEN

AGE IN YEARS	No. OF DEATHS, LUNG CANCER	DEATH RATES			
		Non-smokers	1–14g. [a]	15–24g. [a]	25g. or more
35–54	10	0.00	0.09	0.17	0.26
55–64	24	0.00	0.32	0.52	3.10
65–74	31	0.00	1.35	3.24	4.81
75 or more	19	0.07	2.78	20.7	4.16
All ages	84	0.07	0.47	0.86	1.66

From Doll, R. and Hill, P. B. 1956. Lung cancer and other causes of death in relation to smoking, *Brit. Med. J.* ii:1071–81.
[a] g. = grams of tobacco smoked.

cess, lung cancer for 13.5 per cent, and cancer of other sites for 13.5 per cent.

Subsequently, the past decade has witnessed similar studies by Dorn (1959) for the United States Public Health Service; by Best, Josie, and Walker (1961) for the Canadian Department of National Health and Welfare; and a review of studies on cigarette smoking and health by the California State Department of Public Health (1963). The findings of all these various surveys were similar considering the variegated population and age groups involved and, in general, they were comparable to the results of Doll and Hill and Hammon and Horn. There have been similar points of view expressed by authoritative medical bodies from many parts of the world besides the United States and England.

With this mass of opinion in back of them, chemists began to study this relationship in the laboratory and have isolated at least a dozen carcinogenetic chemicals of a hydrocarbon type from tobacco smoke. It is now suspected that the action of these chemicals is enhanced by phenols and other co-carcinogens and that tobacco smoke may contain yet more carcinogens. Bronchiogenic carcinoma of the lung may not have been produced in animals, but this argument begins to lose some of its weight when it is pointed out that no laboratory animal so far has been trained to smoke cigarettes in the way man does, let alone continue this habit for twenty years.

At this point, we can assemble and review dissenting opinions in the manner in which the American Cancer Society has done in its pamphlet *Cigarette Smoking and Cancer* a booklet published in 1963 that sets forth the evidence on which the society has

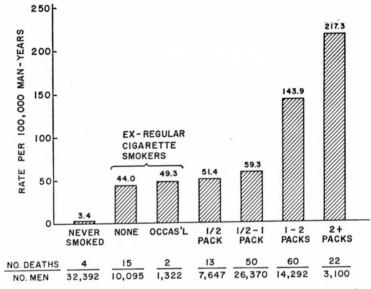

FIG. 41. Age-standardized death rates due to verified cases of broncho-genic carcinoma (exclusive of adenocarcinoma) as compared with the number of cigarettes smoked daily. (From Hammond and Horn, 1958, *J. A. M. A.* 166:1295.)

based its position and its programs. Eight such opinions have been presented here ranging all the way from the statement that since the cause of cancer is unknown, it cannot be said that cigarette smoking is responsible for lung cancer; to indications that the evidence is only statistical and therefore inconclusive; to the conjecture that there may be a common genetic factor conducive to making people smoke and also causing lung cancer. These points deserve investigation. But what is hardly worth investigating is the completely negative attitude taken by some toward the smoking theory, namely, that it simply cannot be.

Although it is well over two years since the report of the U.S. Surgeon General's Committee appeared, a substantial fraction of medical scientists have refused to accept the evidence; certainly a huge fraction of the smoking public in the United States has refused to change its smoking habits as a result of this report, but that is beside the point in this discussion. No doubt a great number of individuals found it too difficult to give up smoking and, after an abortive attempt, returned. Apart from the effect of the report on the smoking habits of the U.S. public, the fact remains that some medical scientists have shown a peculiar resistance to the idea of accepting this etiology.

It would seem that through leads established by the use of statistical methods, evidence of a connection between excessive cigarette smoking and bronchiogenic carcinoma has been established. To the long list of previously known carcinogens, this discovery adds another that is particularly important in view of the way it touches the lives of many of us.

BIBLIOGRAPHY

BAUER, J. T. 1938. A review of the primary carcinomas of the lungs and pleurae occurring in six thousand consecutive necropsies. *Bull. Ayer Clin. Lab.* 3 (No. 15): 139–88.

BEST, E. W. R., JOSIE, G. H., and WALKER, C. B. 1961. A Canadian study of mortality in relation to smoking habits, a preliminary report. *Canadian J. Public Health* 52:99–106.

Cigarette smoking and cancer. 1963. New York: American Cancer Society.

Cigarette smoking and health. 1963. A review of studies by the California State Department of Health. San Francisco: California State Board of Health.

DOLL, R. and HILL, A. B. 1950. Smoking and carcinoma of the lung. Preliminary report. *Brit. Med. J.* 2:739.

DOLL, R. and HILL, A. B. 1956. Lung cancer and other causes of death in relation to smoking: a second report on the mortality of British doctors. *Brit. Med. J.* 2:1071–81.

DORN, C. F. 1959. Tobacco consumption and mortality from cancer and other diseases. Public Health Reports. **74** no. 4. Washington, D.C. Government Printing Office.

HAMMOND, E. C. and HORN, D. 1958. Smoking and death rates: report on 44 months of follow-up of 187,783 men. Part I. Total mortality. Part II. Death rates by cause. *J.A.M.A.* **166**: 1159–72; 1294–1308.

LOMBARD, H. L. and DOERING, C. R. 1928. Cancer studies in Massachusetts. Habits, characteristics and environment of individuals with and without cancer. *New Engl. J. Med.* 198:481–87.

PEARL, R. 1938. Tobacco smoking and longevity. *Science* 87:216–17.

SHIMKIN, M. B. 1964. Science and cancer. Public Health Service Publication No. 1162. Washington, D.C.: U.S. Government Printing Office.

SLOCUMB, J. C. and MACMAHON, B. 1963. Changes in mortality rates from leukemia in the first five years of life. *New Engl. J. Med.* 268:922–25.

Smoking and health. 1964. *A report by a special committee appointed by the Surgeon General of the U.S. Public Health Service.* U.S. Department of Health, Education, and Welfare. Washington, D.C.: Government Printing Office.

WEAVER, W. 1960. The disparagement of statistical evidence. *Science* 123:1859.

WYNDER, E. L. 1961. An appraisal of the smoking-lung cancer issue. *New Engl. J. Med.* 264:1235–40.

Appendixes

Medical Certification of Cause of Death

Because mortality statistics are so widely used as a measure of disease prevalence, it is valuable for the epidemiologist to know the circumstances under which various diagnoses are recorded on these certificates. In the United States there are two parts for entry of the causes of death. Part I relates to the sequence of events that led to death. In Part II are listed any other significant conditions that unfavorably influenced the course of the terminal illness and contributed to the fatal outcome but were not related to the disease or conditions directly causing death. The physician is faced with a decision that may seem easy, but often it is one requiring a high degree of clinical judgment. For guidance in this matter physicians may be referred to recent directions published by the National Office of Vital Statistics, Public Health Service and to other sources of information.[1]

DEFINITIONS

Part I calls for a definitive diagnosis of the cause of death. This is the morbid condition or disease process, abnormality, injury, or poisoning leading directly, or indirectly, to death. These are listed on line *a* (see below).

Symptoms or modes of dying, such as respiratory failure, heart failure, asthenia, and so forth, are not considered to be causes of

[1] *International classification of disease adapted for indexing hospital records by disease and operations.* 1962. Department of Health, Education and Welfare. Washington, D.C.: Government Printing Office.
Physician's handbook on death and birth registration. 1958. 11th ed. U.S. Public Health Service. Washington, D.C.: Government Printing Office.
Medical certification of causes of death. 1960. U.S. Public Health Service. Publication No. 44. Washington, D.C.: Government Printing Office.

death for statistical purposes. If there are antecedent conditions leading to death, these are reported on lines *b* and *c*. Any disease or injury that initiated the train of morbid events leading directly to death or the circumstances of the accident or violence producing fatal injury is indicated here.

Part II records any contributory factors, such as debilitating chronic illness, sensory limitation, or temporary incapacities. Two examples can be given that tell their own story, etiologically speaking.

Part I. (*a*) Cerebral embolus
      (*b*) Arteriosclerotic heart disease
Part II. Inactive pulmonary tuberculosis

Part I. (*a*) Fracture of skull
      (*b*) Trauma from fall
Part II. Pregnancy

The physician's opinion in making these interpretations is very important. In the United States, prior to 1948, whenever multiple causes were entered on the certificate, a clerk using a set of rules selected the one to be used for statistical purposes as the cause of death. Now it is the physician who is asked to give his judgment; this will obviously affect mortality rates for various diseases materially.

Recording Perinatal Deaths

INFANT MORTALITY

The significance of accurate records of infantile deaths has received considerable attention in previous pages. The definition of this rate is the number of deaths that occur during the first year of life per 1,000 live births per year.

Neonatal mortality. This represents deaths in infants during the first month of life. The neonatal death rate is expressed as so many deaths that occur in the first 28 days of life per 1,000 live births per year.

Fetal deaths. For deaths that occur just before birth or just after, this is a more useful designation than the older term "stillbirth." The fetal death rate is the number of fetal deaths occurring in a population during a given year divided by the number of live births in the same year, multiplied by 1,000 to give a working figure. Some investigators have suggested combining data on late fetal and early infantile deaths to obtain a perinatal death rate, but there is no general agreement about the exact range of this period.

Guides for Planning Serologic Surveys

The procedures recommended here represent what may well amount to a major research project. The value of a survey of this type should be weighed against the cost of carrying it out. Such surveys are particularly indicated, nevertheless, in areas where vital statistics on disease prevalence are not available and where periodic samplings of the population are desirable because the immunization status needs to be checked.

ANTIBODY TESTS

The use of any group of serum samples to be tested for antibodies for epidemiologic purposes demands not only a certain degree of knowledge of the population involved but a knowledge of the techniques of the serological tests being used. There should be an appreciation of the degree of the specificity of the tests and some information about the persistence of the antibody in human blood at various levels after one or more infections (or immunization procedures) with a given agent (or antigen). In addition, decisions should be made about what is arbitrarily to be called positive, and, if quantitative determinations are to be made, what is to be considered a high, medium, or low titer. In other words, each antibody and the test for it, whether the end point be demonstrated by a neutralization or a complement-fixing technique, by precipitin or agglutination, hemagglutination or hemagglutination-inhibition reaction, is a special case in itself. Such tests should be carried out according to sufficiently standardized methods so that the work of one laboratory can be compared to that of another, and their limits of error should be known. We will not take time here to particularize about recommended techniques for carrying out various antibody tests. The reader is referred to current editions of textbooks for these technical details.

BLOOD COMPONENTS OTHER THAN ANTIBODIES

As has been mentioned in the chapter on serological epidemiology serum antibodies may have represented the major concern of epidemiologists in the past but they by no means are a measure of the extent to which the serum survey can be utilized. Other fields to be explored have been reviewed in Chapter XII and also have received attention in a WHO Expert Committee Report on Immunologic and Haematologic Surveys which was issued in 1959.[1] The fields mentioned include estimations of blood groups, hemoglobin levels and types of hemoglobins, items of nutritional interest, serum proteins, serum lipids such as cholesterol and triglycerides, and serum enzymes such as pepsin.

Such surveys generally require the services of a team which is oriented to a particular clinical specialty. They may require a much more intimate study of the population to be made and more time to be spent in the field. Also they may require that the blood or serum be preserved in a special way, the latter being stored at temperatures lower than $-20°$ C. Such arrangements must be made well in advance of any expedition in which this type of study is to be done.

POPULATION SAMPLING METHODS

In carrying out serum surveys, it is fundamental to know as much as possible about the character of the population being sampled. In general, the blood specimens should be obtained from normal individuals sampled in a random manner, in adequate numbers, from various age groups, and in special designated areas, which will be defined presently. In particular, infants (from birth to five years) should be included. Only those individuals should be included who are truly representative of the local community, that is, not visitors or newcomers.

[1] *Immunological and haematological surveys. Report of a study group.* 1959. Technical Report Series No. 181. Geneva: World Health Organization.

For random sampling, such procedures as choosing the members of every twentieth or every one-hundredth family in a district might be ideal, but there are obvious limiting factors that render this wholly impractical in most communities. Some compromises must therefore be reached, the various kinds of compromises depending upon local circumstances.

Over and above random serum sampling of a population within a given city or area, one can sometimes divide the population into different sections and determine individual rates for each designated population. Furthermore, a contemporary local census (even though rough) might be desirable, with a view to designating the size of population groups in urban, semiurban, and rural locations, as well as the size of racial segments of the population and of socioeconomic groups.

SOURCES OF CANDIDATES FOR SAMPLING

Assuming from the start that the people are normal individuals and the population from whom blood is taken is chosen in as random a manner as possible, the following groups may prove acceptable provided it is known how much bias is introduced into the collection as a whole. The sources of such populations are several: (1) schools; (2) accident rooms and hospitals; (3) well-baby clinics, or special clinics, that are not attended by those with infectious diseases; (4) institutions of various kinds; (5) military or industrial units; (6) blood donors to a blood bank; and (7) occasionally whole villages, when response to a request for an antibody survey of all age groups happens to be favorable and representative.

AGE DISTRIBUTION

Prior to any serological survey, it is wise to accumulate information about the age composition of the population. This in turn should be related to the eventual sampling system chosen so that one can estimate the degree to which the age groups sampled reflect the actual existing proportions of age groups in the population.

If an extensive short-term sampling of a given population of roughly 120,000 is planned, it is suggested that ideally about 350 sera be collected, perhaps with the breakdown in Table 12. Should various groups of the population each deserve a separate survey on an age-distributional basis, this will multiply the size of the series by as many times as there are groups to be included. Although the ideal of about 350 samples of blood for each group is not an essential, it becomes evident that the investigator

TABLE 12

NUMBER OF SAMPLES RECOMMENDED
FOR EACH AGE GROUP

Age Groups	Number of Samples
0–1	25
1	25
2	25
3	25
4	25
5–9	40
10–14	40
15–19	35
20–29	40
30–39	30
40 and older	40
Total samples of sera	350

should determine at the earliest opportunity what the age groups are and which are likely to deviate in their antibody pattern from the mean and which are more likely to serve his purpose best.

LONGITUDINAL SURVEYS

In longitudinal surveys, the ideal is to obtain so-called matched samples of blood from the same individual collected at intervals of months or years and correlated, if possible, with a record of illness covering the contemporary period. This approach is obviously more informative than the so-called spot survey but much more difficult and time-consuming. Its aim is to relate the frequency of overt and recorded illness to the development of detectable traces of infection in the form of

Appendix II

antibodies and to measure the rise or decline of antibody levels in the same individual. To achieve this end, it is necessary to sample the population of designated areas periodically, at which times medical histories are taken.

The longitudinal approach can be used to advantage when a population is about to be subjected to a change in environment. This applies to military units going overseas or itinerant industrial units, in the event that matched samples can be obtained before departure and after return.

TESTING SAMPLES

It is desirable that the tests involved should be inexpensive ones and adequate facilities for accomplishing the laboratory work should be readily available. The employment of micro methods has some desirable features, particularly when a large number of tests are to be done on each sample of sera and volume of the individual sera is scanty.

As has been repeatedly pointed out by those who have engaged in this work, the simplest part of the program may be the mechanical collection of the sera. The proper testing of a collection of sera, large enough to meet the demands of statistical adequacy, may be a long and most difficult business, so that the simpler the tests used, the better. Statistical analyses and interpretations of the findings, furthermore, require epidemiologic and other kinds of judgment particularly when questions of specificity arise.

COLLECTION, SHIPMENT, AND STORAGE OF SERUM SAMPLES

An attempt should be made to collect from each individual by venipuncture at least 15 or 20 ml. of whole blood, except from children when less may be acceptable. "Vacutainers" have proved useful for this. The addition of anticoagulants or chemical preservatives is not recommended. Another method that is sometimes useful, particularly in the case of young children, is the collection of blood on small filter paper discs; or even on filter paper that when dried can be cut into squares which may serve as aliquots. This relatively crude method is valuable under certain

290

circumstances. The discs or squares can be transported in a dried state in an envelope very inexpensively and do not require refrigeration.[1]

Whole blood, however, should be quickly removed to the laboratory and the serum separated there aseptically, preferably within 24 hours. If serum is to be stored awaiting prompt shipment, this should be done at refrigerator temperature ($+4°$ C). When dry ice is available, serum to be shipped should be by air express with explicit directions that it be picked up on arrival. If dry ice is not available, short-term shipments may be made at refrigerator temperature, or as a last resort, at room temperature. Under field conditions, it may be useful to have a container with liquid nitrogen available, but instructions should be given to all those using this substance.

In the base laboratory, each serum sample can be divided into 0.5 ml. aliquots and then stored in glass ampules. These aliquots can be lyophilized or stored frozen in a ($-20°$ C) freezer depending upon available facilities and on the character of the antibodies or blood components to be studied and the speed at which the tests can be made. If the serum is kept frozen for over six months, a temperature of at most $-15°$ to $-20°$ C should be maintained or lyophilization should be used. The practice of thawing and refreezing the serum apparently does not make for good preservation of certain antibodies. If, however, blood lipids are to be measured, lyophilization is not recommended.

And last, but not least, individual sera with the corresponding personal data and the results of laboratory tests, should be put on IBM punch cards, and, if possible, subjected to computer analyses, if one is to save oneself an immense amount of time-consuming labor.

[1] R. H. Green and E. M. Opton. 1960. *Am. J. Hygiene* **72**: 195–203.

Index

Index

Index

Hippocrates
  interpretation of epidemics, 13, 14
Hippocratic method, 19
Hirsch, August, 5, 130, 255
Horn, D., 276, 277, 278
Host factors in disease, 52
  genetic, 52, 65
  in resistance to, 53
Host susceptibility, 64, 65, 67, 109, 119
Hunter, John, 7, 238
Huntington, Ellsworth, 131

IBM punch cards, 291
Illness rates
  methods of listing, 78
Immune status, tests for, 119, 120, 121
Immunity, inherent, 65, 66
Immunity, measurements of, 119, 128
Immunologic surveys, 125, 126, 128
Increase in use of cigarettes, 274, 276
Increase of lung cancer, 275
Incubation period
  effect on epidemic curve in different diseases, 89–92
Industrial medicine, 150, 151
Infant mortality, 284
Infantile paralysis
  see Poliomyelitis
Infectious disease
  control of, 49, 50
  curtailment, 105
  development of germ theory, 27
  early views of, 49, 50
  etiologic agents in, 49
  importance of host in, 27
  philosophy of, 6
  and serum surveys, 123–27
  in remote places, 133
Infectious hepatitis
  see Hepatitis, infectious
Influenza
  Eskimo epidemic, 132, 136
Insect vectors, 138, 139, 221, 224, 227
International Classification of Disease, 73, 283

International Committee on Nutrition for National Defense, 126
Ischemic heart disease
  age-specific rates, 246
  blood sugar in, 243
  body weight in, 243
  cholesterol in, 244, 248, 249
  and cigarette smoking, 245, 248
  and diabetes, 244, 247
  diagnostic terminology, 237
  diet in, 243, 248
  genetic factors, 244, 245
  and human physique, 247
  hyperlipemia, 244, 247
  and hypertension 244, 250
  incidence, 237
  in Italians, 245
  in Jews, 245
  job classification in, 242
  lipids in, 248, 249
  lipoprotein, 243
  multiple cases in family, 245
  in Negroes, 245
  and nervous strain, 250
  in Norway, 249
  and obesity, 244, 250
  and occupation, 249, 250
  pathogenesis of, 244, 250
  and personal habits, 245, 248
  physical activity in, 245, 250
  racial predilection, 245
  ratio males to females, 246
  saturated fats in, 244, 248, 250
  and sedentary occupations, 247
  sex-specific rates, 246
  somatotypes in, 248
  triglycerides in, 244, 247, 249
  and ways of life, 248
  weight gain after age 25, 247

Jenner, Edward, 155

Koch, Robert, 26, 27
Knowelden, J., 172

Landsteiner, K., 179
Leukemia, 260
Leukosarcoma, 260
Life expectancy
  of females, 102
  increasing, 101
  in different parts of the world, 103
  of males, 102

300

Index